Clinical Intelligence

The Big Data Analytics Revolution in Healthcare

An Analytics Framework for Clinical & Business Intelligence

Clinical Data Analytics, Prediction, Prognostics and Decision Analysis

Peter K. Ghavami, PhD

First Edition

2014

Peter K. Ghavami, PhD

Peter.Ghavami@Northwestu.edu

Peter K. Ghavami, PhD
Peter.Ghavami@Northwestu.edu
8226 125th Place, NE
Kirkland, WA 98033

The author and publisher have taken care in preparations of this book, but make no expressed or implied warranty of any kind and assume no responsibility for errors or omissions. No liability is assumed for the incidental or consequential damages in connection with or arising out of the use of the information or designs contained herein.

Keywords: 1. Big Data Analytics, 2. Data warehouse, 3. Business Intelligence, healthcare quality, patient population management

ISBN-13: 978-1500428594

ISBN-10: 1500428590

Cover Image: Sunburst Plot Highlighting Pedigree and Symptoms, from Noblis Team at IEEE VAST 2010 Challenge, Catherine Campbell, PhD, and et.al. Posted at www.cs.umd.edu/hcil/VASTchallenge2010/Entries/148_Noblis_Processing_MC3/index.htm

Clinical Intelligence

The Big Data Analytics Revolution in Healthcare

An Analytics Framework for Clinical & Business Intelligence

Clinical Data Analytics, Prediction, Prognostics and Decision Analysis

Peter K. Ghavami, PhD

First Edition

2014

Acknowledgements

This book was only possible as a result of my collaboration with many scientists, doctors, surgeons and clinical researchers who have taught me a tremendous deal about scientific research and more importantly about the value of collaboration. To all of them I owe a huge debt of gratitude.

Peter Ghavami
April 14, 2014

To my beautiful wife, Massi

Contents

Introduction

DATA is the new GOLD. And ANALYTICS is the machinery that mines, molds and mints it. Clinical Intelligence is a set of computer-enabled analytics methods, processes and discipline of extracting and transforming raw clinical data into meaningful insight, new discovery and knowledge that helps make more effective clinical and healthcare decisions. Another definition describes Clinical Intelligence as the discipline of extracting and analyzing healthcare data to deliver new insight about the past performance, current operations and prediction of future events. Clinical Intelligence, builds upon years of medical data analytics, healthcare research, clinical trials and proven statistical methods. But, it adds the new wisdom and techniques brought forward by Big Data Analytics. By combining healthcare data analysis, decision analysis, optimization models and prediction algorithm, Clinical Intelligence promises to improve decision making related to quality of care, patient safety, outcomes and cost of care.

Clinical Intelligence is gaining importance not just for improving patient care outcomes or clinical processes; it certainly is the new tool to improve quality of care, reduce costs and improve patient population health. But, it's fast becoming a necessity for operational, administrative and even legal reasons. If data analytics trends from other industries penetrate into healthcare industry, increasingly care providers will be held responsible to *know* about their patients' data and medical history. The executives in healthcare will be held responsible and accountable for knowing what their data is telling them. *Not knowing* or claims such as *my data is spread over several Electronic Medical Record (EMR) systems* will no longer be acceptable excuses in the court of law. The courts will argue that if a hospital database contains the data, then it's the responsibility of the individual care providers, doctors, nurses, and hospital administrators to know such data and the knowledge that the data represents. We can expect that Clinical Intelligence -delivering insight from all data across an array databases and multiple dimensions of clinical data related to an individual patient or a population of patients- will become a standard operating procedure across all aspects of care delivery.

We can trace the first use of Clinical Intelligence to the early1850's, to a celebrated English social reformer, statistician and founder of modern nursing, Florence Nightingale[1]. She has gained prominence for her bravery and caring during the Crimean War, tending to wounded soldiers. But her contributions to statistics and use of statistics for improving healthcare were just as impressive. She was the first to use statistical methods and reasoning to prove better hygiene reduces wound infections and consequently soldier fatalities. At some point during the Crimean War, her advocacy for better hygiene reduced the number of fatalities due to infections by 10x. She was a prodigy who helped popularize graphical representation of statistical data and is attributed to have invented a form of pie-charts that we now call polar area diagram.

Clinical intelligence has come a long way since then and is now gaining popularity thanks to eruption of five new technologies: Big Data Analytics, Cloud computing, mobility, social networking and smaller sensors. Each of these technologies is significant in its unique way to how patient care can be improved and how vast amount of data is being generated. Big Data is known by its three key attributes, known as the three V's: Volume, Velocity, and Variety. The world storage volume is increasing at a rapid pace, estimated to double every year. The velocity at which this data is generated is rising fueled by the advent of mobile devices and social networking. In medicine and healthcare, the cost and size of sensors has shrunk, making continuous patient monitoring and data acquisition from a multitude of human physiological systems an accepted practice.

---

[1] Biography.com, http://www.biography.com/people/florence-nightingale-9423539, accessed, Dec 30, 2012

With the advent of smaller, inexpensive sensors and volume of data collected from patients, physicians are challenged with making increasingly analytical decisions from a large set of data that are being collected per patient. This trend is only increasing giving rise to what's known in the industry as the "big data problem": The rate of data accumulation is rising faster than physicians' cognitive capacity to analyze increasingly large data sets to make decisions. The big data problem offers an opportunity for improved predictive analytics and prognostics.

The U.S. Dept. of Health and Human Services, through the auspices of Center for Medicare & Medicaid Services (CMS) provided incentives for hospitals to implement meaningful use and adopt electronic medical records. The meaningful use policy is laying the groundwork for massive amount of digital data accumulation and new opportunities for clinical intelligence and mining of this data. Of the six stages of meaningful use that the government has outlined, currently only a few are at stage 6. But, the number of stage 6 hospitals is increasing rapidly and with it, the volume of quality data reports mandated by the government.

Similar efforts by the UK Governments' NHS[2] Health and Social Care Information Centre has prompted several frameworks for data analytics in order to accurately and properly classify patients and provide Payment by Results (PbR) guidelines. The NHS PbR is comparable to similar reimbursement policy in the US called Pay for Performance (P4P). NHS has embarked on clinical analytics guidelines to provide classification methods for Casemix Classification Principles based on ICD diagnosis and OPCS procedure classifications. NHS has formed a Casemix Design Authority Group to define and develop the rules and criteria for classifications of Healthcare Resource Groups (HRGs). The current version called HRG4 is used for reimbursements in UK since 2009.

In the U.S. it's becoming important to ensure the accurate classification of patient DRG[3] levels and accurately determine the physician performance through patient care outcomes. These two factors are critical to proper reimbursements and success of payment reform in the U.S. Much of the hospitals' hope for financial viability under the Affordable Care Act (ACA) policies or thriving on Accountable Care Organizations (ACO) business models will depend on their skill in clinical intelligence. Those medical institutions that cultivate clinical intelligence tools and skills are likely to emerge as victors; others will lose the competitive race to become victims.

It's reported that on average most large hospitals in the U.S. have accumulated an average of 400 TeraBytes (400TB) to 0.5 PetaBytes (0.5PB) of data by 2013. A few companies now offer healthcare data vaults and warehousing products including Microsoft with its Amalga product. The NoSQL (Not only SQL) and non-relational database movement such as Hadoop, Lucene and Spark offer new data management tools that allow storage and management of large structured and non-structured data sets.

The variety of data is also increasing. The medical data was confined to paper for too long. As governments such as the United States push medical institutions to transform their practice into electronic and digital format, patient data can take diverse forms. It's now common to think of electronic Medical record

---

[2] National Health Service is the public healthcare system of England. It's funded through taxation and is regarded as one of the world's oldest and largest single-payer healthcare systems.

[3] Diagnosis-related Group (DRG) is a classification method to classify severity and complexity of a patient's health condition into one of originally defined 467 groups which is used by CMS to determine the amount of reimbursement for patient care. It was developed by Robert B. Fetter PhD of the Yale school of Management and John D. Thompson, MPH of the Yale School of Public Health, whose work was also adopted originally for the UK Casemix Classification Principles in the 1960s.

(EMR) to include diverse forms of data such as audio recordings, MRI, Ultrasound, computed tomography (CT) and other diagnostic images, videos captured during surgery or directly from patients, color images of burn and wounds, digital images of dental x-rays, waveforms of brain scans, electro cardiogram (EKG) and the list goes on.

The National Quality Forum (NQF)[4] has endorsed 701 different clinical measures as indicators of quality. The diversity of data types can be realized when all these measures are compared and analyzed together. There are three major purposes for these measures: Clinical quality improvement, Accountability and Research. There are two categories of measures: those related to healthcare delivery and the category that deals with population health measures. These measures provide ample opportunities for data mining and clinical intelligence analytics. The Joint Commission has created a similar measurement and reporting system called ORYX in order to maintain reporting alignment with CMS. While these programs call for measurements and reports, the smart hospitals are conducting clinical intelligence analytics on these measurements in order to improve their internal processes, reduce costs, increase productivity, reduce costs and submit correct reimbursement claims.

Big Data is characterized by 3V's: Velocity, Volume and Variety. This underscores the large volume of data that is being collected and stored by our digital society; the rapid pace at which data is generated by consumers, smart devices, sensors and computer; the variety of data formats which in particular in healthcare spans a wide range of data from text to images and waveforms.

IDC[5] predicts that the worldwide volume of data will increase by 50X from 2010 to 2020. The world volume of data will reach 40ZB (Zetta bytes)[6]. The firm predicts that by 2020, 85% of all this data will be new data types and formats. There will be a 15X growth in machine generated data by 2020. The notion of all devices and appliances generating data has led to the idea of the internet of things, where all devices communicate freely with each other and to other applications through the internet. McKinsey & Company predicts that by 2020, Big Data will be one of the five game changers in US economy and 1/3rd of the world data will be generated in the US.

New types of data will include structured and unstructured text. It will include server logs and other machine generated data. It will include data from sensors, smart pumps, ventilators and physiological monitors. It will include steaming data and customer sentiment data about you. It includes social media data including Twitter, Facebook and local RSS feeds about healthcare. Even today if you're a healthcare provider, you must have observed that your patients are tweeting from the bedside. All these varieties of data types can be harnessed to provide a more complete picture of what is happening in delivery of healthcare.

Big data analytics is finding its own rightful platform in healthcare. The Electronic Medical Record (EMR) systems are not designed to process and handle large volumes, velocity and variety of data. Nor are they intended to handle complex analytics operations such as anomaly detection, finding patterns in data, machine learning, building complex algorithms or predictive modeling.

---

[4] National Quality Measure Clearninghouse, Agency for Healthcare Research and Quality (AHRQ), U.S. Department of Health & Human Services.
[5] International Data Corporation (IDC) is a premier provider of research, analysis, advisory and market intelligence services
[6] Each Zetta byte is roughly 1000 Exabytes and each Exabyte is roughly 1000 Petabytes. A Petabyte is about 1000 TeraBytes.

The traditional data warehouse strategies based on relational databases suffer from a latency of up to 24 hours. These data warehouses can't scale quickly with large data growth and because they impose relational and data normalization constraints, their use is limited. In addition, they provide retrospective insight and not real-time or predictive analytics.

EMR is primarily a transactional system taking feeds from source systems and interface engines. A big data analytics platform is needed to take data from EMR and enterprise data warehouses to provide a complete and real time analytics. I predict that healthcare organizations will recognize the importance of investing in a clinical analytics platform as they've invested in EMR systems as a platform.

The value proposition of big data analytics in healthcare is derived from the improvements and balance between cost and outcomes. According to a McKinsey & Company research paper, big data analytics is the platform to deliver five values to healthcare: Right living, Right Care, Right Provider, Right Value, Right Innovation[7]. These new data analytics value systems drive boundless opportunities in improving patient care and population health on one hand and reducing waste and costs on the other.

But medical data analytics is not challenged just by the 3V's. It brings its own unique set of challenges that I call the 4 S's: Situation, Scale, Semantics and Sequence. Taking data measurements from patients has different connotation in different situations. For example, a blood pressure value taken from a patient conveys a different signal to a doctor if the measurement was taken at rest, while standing up or just after climbing some stairs. Scale is a challenge in medicine since certain measurements can vary drastically and yet remain clinically insignificant compared to other measurements that have a limited rate of change but a slight change can be significant. Some clinical variables have a limited range versus others have a wider range For example; analyzing data that contains patient blood pressure and body temperature that have a limited range requires understanding of scale since a slight change can be significant in the analysis of patient outcome. In contrast, a similar amount of fluctuation in patient fluids measured in milliliters may not be a serious. As another example, consider the blood reticulocytes value (rate of red blood cell production). A normal Reticulocyte value should be zero, but a 1% increase is cause for alarm, an indication of body compensating for red blood cell count, a possible body compensation to shock to the bone marrow.

We can see the complexity associated with scale and soft thresholds best in lab blood tests: the normal hemoglobin level in adults is somewhere between 12 to 15 and a drop to 10 a physician might choose to prescribe iron supplements but measured at 4 will require a blood transfusion. There are varying degrees of data thresholds and scales with different lab test results. The blood iron level greater than 350mg/dL is considered acute iron toxicity, but this is soft threshold. Often a soft threshold is perceived differently by different doctors. For example, in pediatrics a child in 90th percentile of weight is considered obese. In pediatrics, the definition of infant "failure to thrive" is does not have concrete and hard thresholds. For example, a child being less than 3rd or 5th percentile in weight in two consequence doctor visits or if the child drops two percentiles in weight fits "failure to thrive". The range of 3rd to 5th percentile can be subject to interpretation and cause of confusion for clinical data analytics. To be more sensitive, the analytics program would select the 5th percentile line instead of 3rd percentile line.

---

[7] "The Big Data Revolution in Healthcare", Center for US Health System Reform, McKinsey & Co. 2013

Semantics are critical to data analytics. As much as 80% of clinical data is non-structured data in form of narrative text or audio recording. Correctly extracting the pertinent terms from such data is a challenge. Tools such as Natural Language Processing (NLP) methods combined with medical libraries such as SNOMED, LOINC and UMLS are used to extract useful data from patient medical records. However, understanding sentence structure and relationships between medical terms are critical to detect the physician's sentiment in the medical record. For example, detecting the indications automatically requires accurate determination if the diagnosis positive or negative, likely or requires follow up tests? Semantics are critical to interpretation of data values since no single data value from a patient tells the entire story about the patient's current health or health history.

For example the blood sodium test might indicate a hypernatremia, a condition of low-sodium. The threshold states that blood sodium level less than 136 mEq/L (Milli equivalents per Liter) is an indicator for low-sodium level. Knowing the context, semantics and scale (thresholds for values) are critical to data analytics in healthcare.

That brings us to the next challenge in clinical intelligence: Sequence. Physiological and clinical data are collected over certain time periods, during a hospital stay or over several years. The values measured during different times are significant and in particular the sequence of those values can have different interpretations. It's important that clinical analytics models allow for time-series analysis, pattern matching and modal interpretations of data.

Despite these challenges, four Big Data analytics technologies are converging to make medical and healthcare data analytics more practical. One clinical analytics company is integrating data analytics, semantic analytics, data visualization and Natural Language Processing to create more powerful platforms for medical data analysis.

This book is divided into three parts. Part I covers the basics of clinical intelligence, big data analytics architecture overview and a framework, plus clinical use cases and analytics-based application opportunities. The basic topics include a review of a 3-phase analytics process: data ingestion and data management, analytics engines and dashboards. It continues to cover medical term extraction, Natural Language processing (NLP), Clinical Prediction Rules (CPR), Clinical Documentation Improvement (CDI), metrics and measurement for improving patient care and safety.

Part II introduces a control theoretic framework to Clinical Intelligence. It covers advanced topics in clinical prediction and prognostics proposing new methods of clinical data analytics. These methods strive to improve accuracy of classification and prediction. Prediction is important because during the course of care, patients frequently develop escalating health problems that lead to medical complications, costly treatments, severe pains, disabilities and even death. Predicting such escalations provides the opportunity to apply preventive measures that result in better patient safety, quality of care and lower medical costs; in short, timely prediction can save lives and avoid further medical complications. Prognostics methods using Artificial Neural Networks (ANN) promise to deliver new insights into future patient health status that provide more effective medical treatment during the patient hospital stay.

Investigation and development of a methodical framework for medical data prognostics in general and use of committee of algorithms in particular have not been adequately explored in prior research in the realms of healthcare and clinical analytics. A framework for prediction of patient health status from clinical data is needed to assist physicians in their clinical decision process. This part investigates and contributes to three essential ideas for improving clinical intelligence and healthcare analytics: 1) A control system approach to prognostics for prediction, 2) A generalized committee of models framework as prognostics engine, and 3) Study the viability of such framework on a particular clinical case.

Part III describes a case study using the proposed framework. It considers issues related to accuracy, specificity and sensitivity in Clinical Intelligence analytics. In this study, the output was defined by a marker called Deep Vein Thrombosis (DVT).

Advances in vital-signs monitoring software/hardware, sensor technology, miniaturization, wireless technology and storage allow recording and analysis of large physiological data in a timely fashion (Yu, Liu, McKenna, et al. 2006). This provides both a challenge and an opportunity. The challenge is that the medical decision maker must sift through vast amount of data to make the appropriate care decision. The opportunity is to analyze this large amount of data in real time to provide forecasts about the health of the patient and assist with clinical decisions.

Leapfrog is one of many organizations that attempt to measure and improve patient safety and outcomes. Leapfrog and several other organizations gather and compare measurements from hospitals across multiple care outcome areas. While most hospitals are working hard to collect and report on these clinical measurements, but soon they'll seek to understand the underlying reasons and root causes of their clinical outcomes. They'll wonder why they're achieving those results and how their results could be better. Finally, they'll wonder what questions they're not asking. Clinical intelligence tools can investigate the root causes of outcomes by determining the underlying factors that are associated with a certain outcome. They promise to bring new insights from data to answer not only complex clinical practice questions but also to tell us which questions we're not asking.

In a survey conducted by Aberdeen Group, several healthcare providers including both inpatient and outpatient facilities where surveyed. The survey found the best-in-class healthcare organizations (those who rank higher on the key performance indicators-KPIs), were much more savvy and familiar with clinical analytics than the lower performing healthcare organizations[8]. In fact, 67% of the best-in-class providers used clinical analytics versus 42% adoption among the low-performing providers. In terms of ability to improve quality, the best-in-class providers using analytics were twice as capable (almost 60% vs. 30%) as the low-performing providers to respond and resolve quality issues. One take away from this research was that healthcare providers who don't use analytics are unable to make the proper process and quality changes because they are simply not aware of the relevant and needed facts and metrics to make those changes.

But we should approach this topic with caution and open eyes, as there are limits to Clinical Intelligence. Clinical Intelligence helps doctors, nurses and hospital administrators and care providers with a heightened sense of awareness, with higher level of knowledge about their patients, with both clinical and situational awareness so they can make more appropriate and effective decisions in their course of work. But, clinical Intelligence does not replace physicians. Using analytics we can classify the data, make predictions and

---

[8] "Healthcare Analytics: Has the Need Ever Been Greater? By David White, Aberdeen Group, A Harte-Hanks Company, September 2012.

provide decision assistance and gain better understanding of patient data. We're able to achieve these analytics insights and useful patterns and predictions to help physicians make better informed decisions. Data analytics alone is not enough to render a treatment. We enable physicians to "see" the data but ultimately physicians need to "see" the patient too. The fact is that physicians don't treat data, they treat patients. In summary, Clinical Intelligence, namely the application of data analytics to patient data needs to serve the care providers in a way that provides meaningful applications and use cases.

Given the rising volume of data and the demand or high-speed data access that can handle analytics some IT leaders are contemplating to invest in dedicated analytics platform. EMR systems are not designed to handle high-speed access to data for analytics and thus are inadequate. As a result specialized data analytics platform is needed to handle high-volume data storage and high-speed access required for analytics.

While Big Data Analytics promises phenomenal improvements in healthcare, as with any technology acquisition we want to take prudent steps towards adoption. We want to gauge Return on Investment (ROI) and define criteria for success. A successful project must demonstrate palpable benefits and value derived from new insights. Implementing Big Data Analytics on clinical data will be necessary and standard procedure for healthcare organizations as they strive to identify any remaining opportunities in improving efficiency, clinical outcomes and cutting costs, the holistic benefits of Clinical Intelligence that I call Return on Analytics (ROA).

As I mentioned in my earlier book, "Lean, Agile and Six Sigma IT Management", success implementation of big data analytics requires team effort and lean approach. Team effort is required because no single vendor or solution satisfies all analytics needs of the organization. Collaboration and partnerships among all user communities in the organization as well as among vendors in needed for successful implementation. Lean approach is required in order to avoid duplication of efforts and systems as well as eliminate wasteful IT investments.

The future of Clinical Intelligence, the application of big data analytics to healthcare data is bright and will be so for many years to come. We're finally able to shed light on the data that have been locked up in the darkness of our electronic systems for years. When you consider other applications of analytics such as precision medicine and genomics data analytics, there are endless opportunities to improve healthcare outcomes and reduce costs using data analytics. So far, medical research has primarily used in-vivo and in-vitro methods for care, but the growth of data analytics will add in-silico as a standard to augment these methods.

Now, let's start our journey through the book.

PART I:

Clinical Intelligence

Chapter 1. Clinical Intelligence

1.1 Clinical Intelligence Definition

Clinical Intelligence is a set of computer-enabled methods, processes and discipline of extracting and transforming raw clinical data into meaningful insight, new discovery and knowledge that helps make more effective clinical and healthcare decisions. This is to be contrasted from Business Intelligence for two reasons: First, Business intelligence (BI) deals with raw business data, typically structured data, and provides insight and information for business decision making. It is used and defined broadly to include business data query and analysis, even including data mining. In contrast Clinical Intelligence deals with clinical data. Second, Clinical Intelligence requires more advanced statistical methods and analytics modeling than BI and often deals with much more complex and unstructured data types.

Clinical Intelligence increasingly deals with vast amount of data -mostly unstructured information stored in a wide variety of mediums and formats- and complex data sets collected through fragmented databases during patients' episodes of care. When using this broad definition, Clinical Intelligence requires data collection, data integration, data transformation, analytical methods, clinical decision support, clinical prediction rules, reporting and dashboards. A broader definition would add data management, data quality, and data warehousing. The high adoption of electronic medical records and digital diagnostic equipment are creating a big data opportunity, making clinical intelligence more relevant and feasible. For the purpose of this book, we'll focus our attention to the first definition.

There are similar challenges yet significant differences between Clinical Intelligence and Business Intelligence. Many of the challenges to get the right Business Intelligence (BI) are the same in getting the right Clinical Intelligence (CI). Business Intelligence has been defined as the ability to understand the relationships of presented facts in such a way to guide action towards a desired goal[9]. This definition could apply to both BI and CI. But on closer examination, their differences are critical to note. One difference is the nature of data and the other is purpose. Business Intelligence provides business insight from raw data for the purpose of enabling strategy, tactics, and business decision making. In contrast Clinical Intelligence strives to provide insight to enable clinical decisions from clinical data which are often ambiguous, incomplete, conditional and inconclusive. The choices among Clinical decisions as we shall discuss are often less clear and subject to debate among clinical specialists. The third difference is that often higher accuracy of analysis is needed to make the right clinical decision. These factors combine to create a complex analytical environment for the clinical intelligence analyst.

Clinical data analytics, answers 3 questions related to the events, workflows, patients, providers and procedures. These questions explains what has happened in the past, what is happening right now and what is about to happen.

The retrospective analytics can explain and present knowledge about the events of the past, show trends and help find root-causes for those events. The real-time analysis shows what is happening right now. It works to present situational awareness, alarms when data reaches certain threshold or send reminders when a certain rule is satisfied. The prospective analysis presents a view in to the future. It attempts to predict what

---

[9] Hans Peter Luhn, "A Business Intelligence System", IBM Journal 2 (4): 314, 1958.

will happen, what are the future values of certain variables. Figure 1.1 shows the taxonomy of the 3 analytics questions.

The Past	The Present	The Future
Retrospective View	**Real-time View**	**Prospective View**
What Happened?	What is Happening now?	What will happen next?
Why it happened?	Uses real-time Data	How can I intervene?
Uses historical Data	Actionable dashboards	Uses historical and real-time Data
Delivers Static dashboards	Alerts	Predictive dashboards
	Reminders	Knowledge-based dashboards

Fig. 1.1 – The 3 temporal questions in healthcare data analysis

1.2 The Distinction between BI and Analytics

The purpose of Business Intelligence (BI) is to transform raw data into information, insight and meaning for business purposes. Analytics is for discovery, knowledge creating, assertion and communication of patterns, associations, classifications and learning from data. While both approaches crunch data and use computers and software to do that, the similarities end there.

With BI, we're providing a snapshot of the information, using static dashboards. We're working with normalized and complete data typically arranged in rows and columns. The data is structured and assumed to be accurate. Often, data that is out of range or outlier are removed before processing. Data processing uses simple, descriptive statistics such as mean, mode and possibly trend lines and simple data projections to extrapolation about the future.

In contrast analytics deals with all types of data both structured and unstructured. In medicine about 80% of data is unstructured in form of medical notes, charts and reports. Analytics does not mandate data to be clean and normalized. In fact, it makes no assumption about data normalization. It can analyze many varieties of data to provide view into patterns and insights that are not humanly possible. Analytics methods are dynamic and provide dynamic and adaptive dashboards. They use advanced statistics, artificial intelligence techniques, machine learning, feedback and natural language processing (NLP) to mine through the data. They detect patterns in data to provide new discovery and knowledge. The patterns have a geometric shape and these shapes as some data scientists believe, have mathematical representations that explain the relationships and associations between data elements.

Unlike BI dashboards that are static and show snapshots of data, analytics methods provide data visualization and adaptive models that are robust to changes in data and in fact learn from changes in data.

While BI uses simple mathematical and descriptive statistics, Analytics is highly model-based. A data scientist builds models from data to show patterns and actionable insight. Feedback and machine learning are concepts found in Analytics. Table 1.1 illustrates the distinctions between BI and Analytics.

Business Intelligence	Analytics
Information from processing raw data	Discovery, Insight, patterns, learning from data
Structured data	Unstructured & Structured data
Simple descriptive statistics	NLP, Classifiers, Machine learning, Pattern Recognition, Predictive modeling, optimization, model-based
Tabular, cleansed & complete data	Dirty data, missing & noisy data, non-normalized data
Normalized data	Non-normalized data, many types of data elements
Data snapshots, static queries	Streaming data, continuous updates of data & models, feedback & auto-learning
dashboards snapshots & reports	Visualization, knowledge discovery

Table 1.1 – The differences between Business Intelligence and Data Analytics

1.3 Why Analytics?

The most common form of Clinical Intelligence has been grounded in linear and descriptive analytics mostly driven by the need for reporting quality measures. But, Clinical Intelligence goes beyond descriptive statistics. While descriptive statistics are important to understanding and gaining insight about data, Clinical Intelligence covers broader and deeper methods to study data and interpret the results. These methods includes machine learning (ML) and non-linear algorithms and as well as the introduction of multi-algorithm approaches.

Traditionally, descriptive statistics answer "what" but offer little help on "why" and "how" (Burke 2012). They are good at making generalizations about one population versus another, but perform poorly on an individual basis. One example of analytics is classification. A descriptive statistics measure might suggest that 65% of patients with certain preconditions to a disease respond to a specific therapy. But, when a patient is diagnosed with the disease how can we determine if the patient is among the 65% of population?

Descriptive statistics look at the past events, but they're not a good method to predict what will happen in the future. Similarly, descriptive statistics offer little insight about causal relationships that help care providers and researchers identify root causes of ailments so they can target and prevent causes from manifesting into full disease. While descriptive analytics are simple tools to determine what is happening in the environment of care, and populations of patients, they come short in giving us the details often necessary to make intelligent care decisions.

Clinical Intelligence can help with patient classifications not just by the traditional demographics such as age, gender and life styles, but by relevant medical and clinical characteristics related to issues, medical conditions, risk propensities, genetic disposition and therapeutic response probabilities.

Clinical Intelligence give us the ability to optimize and tailor the course of care to each individual patient based on multitudes of factors that go into defining the medical protocol of care for such patients: prior medical history, allergies and precautions, personal risk factors, genetic traits, work and life styles, safety management, etc.

Clinical Intelligence gives us the ability to perform multi-factorial analysis to determine the utility (or health value) associated with different courses of care. Such analysis enables care provider to select the right set of personalized care and outcome measures (Burke 2012).

For each patient, there are various indicators associated with medical outcomes. Analytics enables care providers to "see" these indicators including previously over-looked indicators and apply the correct weight (or consideration) to these indicators when making diagnosis and tracking outcomes.

Similarly a great amount of energy and focus is being spent on quality indicators. Analytics can uncover causal relationships between a number of quality indicators and factors that influence or affect those indicators in a patient population or specific patients.

Clinical Intelligence can be used to calculate more accurate measure of patient risk stratification, determining the level of health complication, comorbidity impact and how serious a patient's health status will affect the outcomes. From such calculations, risk profiles about patients can be determined which will help in designing care plans for a population of patients with the same profiles. This type of classification is helpful to Accountable Care Organization (ACO) plans and pricing.

Analytical tools in medicine are able to suggest clinical care plans and protocol pathways with corresponding prediction for outcomes. Such tools are able to provide tradeoffs between complementary care options, conflicting care scenarios, risk management and help with the selection of the most optimal care pathways.

Clinical Intelligence has a prominent place in continuous improvement of care and processes. By true understanding of relationships in large data sets, we're able to track and identify underlying relationships between process activities and the outcomes, quality, cost, complications and safety. The assumption is that the data is being collected and stored on a day-to-day and even minute to minute as the new electronic medical records and electronic medical devices are increasingly capable of record events and records through the patients' course of care.

Analyzed data provides a great source for feedback for processes where data was collected from. A faster feedback provides a tighter feedback loop that translates into higher control over processes. Gone are the days when staff would pour over data in Business Intelligence systems over months. Today, Clinical Intelligence is capable of providing insight into your operations in real time.

The most recent Clinical Intelligence advances in coding and reimbursement are enabling hospitals to more accurately gauge the patient risk, complications, Diagnostic Related Group (DRG) values and avoid under-coding and under documentation, resulting in higher reimbursement from insurance payers.

In a survey conducted by vendor research firm KLAS Enterprises, nearly 56% of organizations surveyed are moving to an enterprise strategy for BI use (Gillespie 2011). The report indicates that many enterprises are adopting strategic BI solutions so because they're tired of having internal arguments about data."(KLAS 2011)

The key barrier to providing consistent data reports across the enterprise in healthcare is typically due to the distributed and fragmented nature of information systems. By creating data warehouses and BI systems including Microsoft's Amalga, Epic's Clarity and McKesson's HBI, also McKesson's TIBCO Spotfire or IBM's Cognos, healthcare institutions are hoping to normalize their data across their system of care. Other leading providers of analytics applications, Caradigm, Lumedix, Dimension Insight, Information Builders, Explorys, Health Catalyst, Predixion, and Apixio are blazing the trail of analytics and prediction.

However, there are many challenges related to the format, meaning and scale of data. To compound the problem, much of the data is unstructured, in form of free text in reports, charts and even scanned documents. There is a lack of enterprise wide dictionary of data terms, units of measure and frequency of reporting.

As one medical officer mentioned, recording and later analyzing patients' blood pressure is not as easy as taking the measurements. It's quite relevant to know patient's position, whether the measurement was taken when the patient was lying in bed, sitting or standing as the values and interpretation of values are significantly different.

Currently, almost half of BI analysis are performed by niche applications such as those targeted for Emergency Dept.(ED) or Operating Room (OR). Their advantage is the specialized BI reports customized to the niche line of care. However, the trend is shifting towards enterprise wide BI applications (KLAS 2011).

Increasingly going forward, the Clinical Intelligence tools of choice can perform three important tasks: Discover, Detect, Distribute. The leading Clinical Intelligence solutions will discover data across disparate and fragmented datasets that reside in various medical, administrative and financial systems. Second, it can aggregate such data –often in real time- normalize and index data on demand. Then perform analytics on the data including semantic analysis through Natural Language Processing (NLP). Finally, it must be able to distribute some actionable insights to user devices, often mobile devices carried by users such as physicians and other care providers.

In a survey of 256 decision makers at health insurance companies, hospitals and health systems surveyed in 2013[10]: 66% indicated they are excited about the future potential of Big Data analytics, 87% agreed that Big Data is an important development that will have at least some impact on their business in the future. Of the respondents, 84% expressed difficulty finding staff that can synthesize complex data sets and glean actionable information from them.

- [10] http://www.hitconsultant.net/2013/12/05/2-roadblocks-to-realization-of-big-data-in-healthcare/

1.4 Analytics Platform Framework

When considering building analytics tools and applications, a data analytics strategy and governance is recommended. One of the strategies is to avoid implementing point-solutions that are stand-alone applications and do not integrate with other analytics applications. Consider implementing an analytics platform that supports many analytics applications and tools integrated in the platform. A 4-layer framework is proposed here as the foundation for the entire enterprise analytics applications. The 4-layer framework consists of a data management layer, an analytics engine layer and a presentation layer as shown in the Figure 1.2-A.

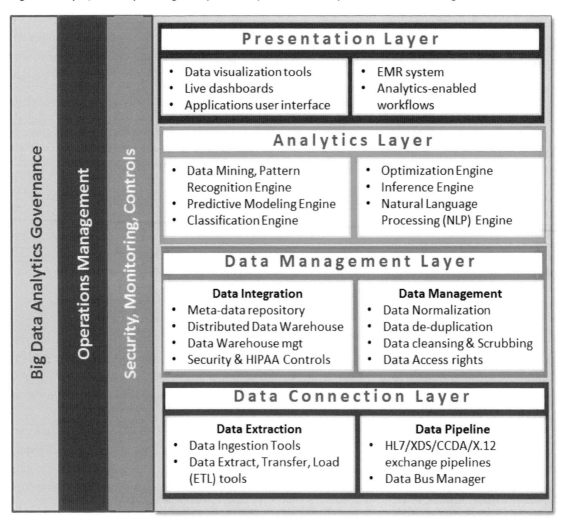

Fig 1.2-A – The 4-layer Data Analytics Framework

In practice, you'll make choices about what software and vendors to adopt for building this framework. The layers are color coded to match a data-bus architecture shown in Figure 1.2-B. The data management layer (in blue color) includes the distributed or centralized data repository. This framework assumes that the modern enterprise data warehouses will consist of distributed and networked data warehouses.

The analytics layer (in green color) may be implemented using SAS and R statistical language or solutions from other vendors who provide the analytics engines in this layer.

The presentation layer (in red color) may consist of various visualization tools such as Tableau, QlikView, or McKesson SpotFire, and other clinical applications including the EMR system. Architecturally, your EMR system belongs to this layer. In a proper implementation of this framework, the EMR offers analytics-driven workflows and therefore tight integration between the EMR system and the other two layers (data and analytics) are critical to successful implementation.

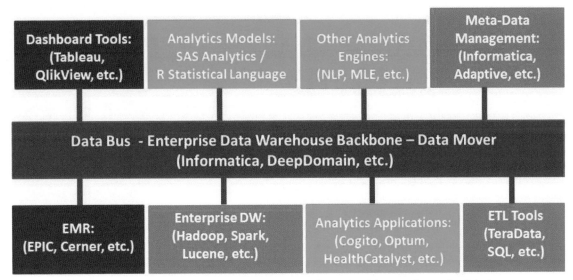

Fig 1.2-B – The Enterprise Data Bus Architecture Schematic with Example Vendor Solutions

Some notes and explanations for Fig 1.2-B are necessary. The references to vendor and product names are by no means an endorsement of these products. They're only provided as illustration as the reader is encouraged to perform their own research and comparative analysis to build their data analytics infrastructure. The analytics engines referenced here include NLP (Natural Language Processing) and MLE (Machine Learning Engine), but there are other engines that the organization can obtain or build to perform specific, targeted analytics functions.

1.5 Data Connection layer

In the data Connection layer, data analysts set up data ingestion pipelines and data connectors to access data. They might apply methods to identify meta-data in all source data repositories. This layer starts with making an inventory of where the data is created and stored. The data analysts might implement Extract, Transfer, and Load (ETL) software tools to extract data from their source. Often in healthcare, the sources of data include Electronic Medical Record (EMR) systems, Financial and Billing systems, Employee time keeping, patient ADT (Admit, Discharge, Transfer) systems and other inpatient or outpatient clinical information systems. The data extraction might use HL7 or variants of HL7 in XML format or CCDA/XDS standards for data transfer. Other data exchange standards such as X.12 might be used to transfer data to the Data Management Layer.

1.6 Data Management layer

Once the data has been extracted, data scientist must perform a number of functions that are grouped under data management layer. The data may need to be normalized and stored in certain database architectures to improve data query and access by the analytics layer. We'll cover taxonomy of database tools including SQL, NoSQL, Hadoop, Shark and other architecture in the upcoming sections.

In this layer, we must pay attention to HIPAA standards for security and privacy. The data scientist will use the tools in this layer to apply security controls, such as those from HITRUST (Health Information Trust Alliance). HITRUST offers a Common Security Framework (CSF) that aligns HIPAA security controls with other security standards.

Data Scientists may apply other data cleansing programs in this layer. They might write tools to de-duplicate (remove duplicate records) and resolve any data inconsistencies. Once the data has been ingested, it's ready to be analyzed by engines in the next layer.

Since big data requires fast retrieval several organizations, in particular the open source foundation have developed alternate database architectures that allow parallel execution of queries, read, write and data management.

There are three architectural taxonomies or strategies for storing big data that impact data governance, management and analytics:

1. Analyze Data in-Place: Most data analysts use the native application and SQL query on the application's data without moving the data. Many data analysts systems build analytics solutions on top of an application's database without using data warehouses. They perform analytics in place, from the existing application's data tables without aggregating data into a central repository. The analytics that are offered by EMR companies as integrated solutions to their EMR system fits this category.

2. Build Data Repository: Another strategy is to build data warehouses to store all the enterprise data in a central repository. These central repositories are often known as Enterprise Data Warehouse (EDW). Data from EMR system(s), clinical information systems, financial and operations systems are normalized and stored in these data warehouses. The data is either collected through ETL extraction (batch files) or via interface engines. Data Warehouses have four limitations: they often lag behind the real time data by as much as 24 hours; that they apply relational database constraints to data which adds to the complexity of data normalization; their support for diverse, new data types is nascent; and they're difficult to use and slow to handle data analytics search and computations. Variations of this architecture include Parallel Data Warehouses (PDW) and Distributed Data Warehouses (DDW).

3. Pull Data on-Demand: An alternate approach is to build an on-demand data pull. This schema leaves the data in the original form on the application and only pulls the data when it's needed for analysis. This approach adopted by only a few hospitals utilizes an external database that maintains pointers to where the data resides in the source system. The external data base keeps track of all data and data dictionaries. When an analytics application requires a piece of data, the external databases pulls the data from the source system on demand and discards it when done.

Most analytics models require access to the entire data because often they annotate the data with tags and additional information which are necessary for models to perform. However, the modern architectures use a networked data warehouse model using a data warehouse data-bus model that embody and network all sources of data (as shown in Figure 1.2-B). The Data-Bus connects the sources of data to the analytics tools and the user-facing applications and dashboards. Increasingly, EMR systems will serve analytics-driven dashboards and actionable workflows while they rely on other components for analytics. The Data-Bus diagram in Figure 1.2B demonstrates a networked architecture scenario for an enterprise. In this scenario, the EMR system is color coded in red, along with the dashboard tools as indication of presentation layer components. The meta-data manager and cloud services are color coded in blue to convey they belong to data management layer. The analytics tools in this scenario are provided by SAS and by R Statistical language. However, your Data-Bus architecture components may vary depending on your pre-exiting infrastructure and data warehouse components.

The traditional data management approaches have adopted centralized data warehouse architectures. The traditional data warehouses, namely a central repository, or a collection of data from disparate applications have not been as successful as expected. One reason is that data warehouses are expensive and time consuming to build. The other reason is that they are often limited to structured data types and difficult to use for data analytics, in particular when unstructured data is involved. Finally, traditional data warehouses insist on relational data base and tabular structures and data to be normalized. Such architectures are too slow to handle the large volume of data queries required by data analytics models. They require normalized relations between tables and data elements.

Star Schema: The more advanced data warehouses have adopted Kimbal's Star Schema or Snowflake Schema to overcome the normalization constraints. The Star schema splits the business process into Fact tables and Dimension tables. Fact tables describe measurable information about entities while Dimension tables store attributes about entities. The Star schema contains one or more Fact tables reference any number of Dimension tables. The logical model typically puts the Fact table in the center and the Dimension tables surrounding it, resembling a star (hence the name). Snowflake schema is similar to Star schema but its tables are normalized.

Star schemas are denormalized data where normalization rules, typical of transactional relational databases, are relaxed during design and implementation. This approach offers simpler and faster queries and access to cube data. However they share the same disadvantage with the non-SQL data bases (discussed below), the rules of data integrity are not strongly enforced.

Non-SQL Database schema: In order to liberate data from relational constraints, several alternate architectures have been devised in the industry as explained in the next sections. These non-traditional architectures include methods that store data in a columnar fashion, or store data in distributed and parallel file systems while others use simple but highly scalable tag-value data structures. The more modern big data storage architectures are known by names like NoSQL, Hadoop, Cassandra, Lucene, SOLR, Shark and other commercial adaptations of these solutions.

NoSQL database means Not Only SQL. A NoSQL database provides storage mechanism for data that is modeled other than the tabular relations constraint of relational databases like SQL Server. The data structures are simple and designed to meet the specific types of data, so the data scientist has the choice of selecting the best fit architecture. The database is structured either in a tree, columnar, graph or key-value pair. However, a NoSQL database can support SQL-like queries.

Hadoop is an open-source database framework for storing and processing large data sets on low-cost, commodity hardware. Its key components are the Hadoop distributed file systems (HDFS) for storing data over multiple servers and MapReduce for processing the data. Written in Java and developed at Yahoo, Hadoop stores data with redundancy and speeds-up searches over multiple servers. Commercial versions of Hadoop include HortonWorks and Cloudera.

Cassandra is another open-source distributed database management system designed to handle large data sets at higher performance. It provides redundancy over distributed server clusters with no single point of failure. Developed at Facebook to power the search function at higher speeds, Cassandra has a hybrid data structure that is a cross between a column-oriented structure and key-value pair. In the key-value pair structure, each row is uniquely identified by a row key. The equivalent of a RDBMS table is stored as rows in Cassandra where each row includes multiple columns. But, unlike a table in an RDBMS, different rows may have different set of columns and a column can be added to a row at any time.

Lucene is an open-source database and data retrieval system that is especially suited for unstructured data or textual information. It allows full text indexing and searching capability on large data sets. It's often used for indexing large volumes of text. Data from many file formats such as .pdfs, HTML, Microsoft Word, and OpenDocument can be indexed by Lucene as long as their textual content can be extracted.

SOLR is a high speed, full-text search platform available as an open-source (Apache Lucene project) program. It's highly scalable offering faceted search and dynamic clustering. SOLR (pronounced "solar") is reportedly the most popular enterprise search engine. It uses Lucene search library as its core and often is used in conjunction with Lucene.

Hive is another open-source Apache project designed as a data warehouse system on top of Hadoop to provide data query, analysis and summarization. Developed initially at Facebook, it's now used by many large content organizations include Netflix and Amazon. It supports a SQL-like query language called HiveQL. A key feature of Hive is indexing to provide accelerated queries, working on compressed data stored in Hadoop database.

Spark is a modern data analytics platform, a modified version of Hadoop. Its built on the notion that distributed data collections can be cached in memory across multiple cluster nodes for faster processing. Spark fits into the Hadoop distributed file system offering 10 times (for in-disk queries) to 100 times (in-memory queries) faster processing for distributed queries. It offers tools for queries distributed over in-memory cluster computers that allow applications run repeated in-memory queries rapidly. Spark is well suited to certain applications such as machine learning (which will be discussed in the next section).

Shark is a distributed SQL query system for Hadoop data. It offers higher query performance and Hive compatibility. Shark is the ideal query system for Spark platform. On certain applications, for example, on performing logistic regression analysis when the same data items are needed for computation, Shark provides in-memory access resulting in faster processing.

Real-time vs. Batch Analytics: Many of the traditional business intelligence and analytics happen on batch data; a set of data is collected over time and the analytics is performed on the batch of data. In contrast real-time analysis refers to techniques that update information and perform analysis at the same rate as they receive data. Real-time analysis enables timely decision making and control of systems. With real-time analysis, data and results are continuously refreshed and updated.

Data Aggregation & Warehousing: Healthcare institutions are replete with disparate databases and data spread all over the firm. Some hospitals and healthcare organizations have accumulated as many as hundreds, perhaps close to a thousand of Access databases, several SQL servers, diverse files stored in various file shares in file servers and plus files in Sharepoint or similar content management system. While implementing data warehouses have been useful to consolidate data, not all of these data files are found in a common data warehouses. Hospital managers, physicians and quality assurance staff would like to run analytics across these vast and diverse data storage repositories without having to create a massive data base. As part of data governance activity, the organization must take an inventory of its data warehouses, sources of data and uses of data. The diagram below (Figure 1.4) shows an example of a data eco-system developed at a healthcare system to capture a single-view of their databases and application inventory.

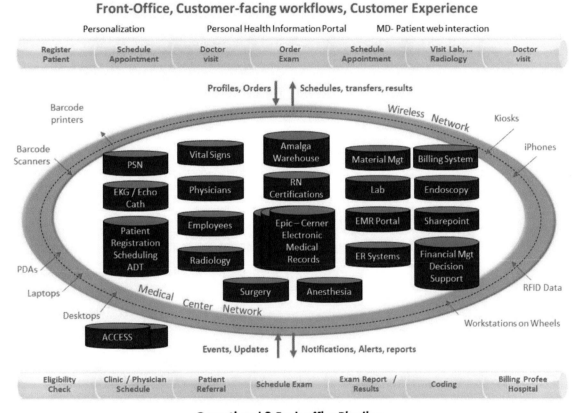

Fig. 1.3 - Enterprise View of Data Eco-system at a Healthcare System

Ultimately, the goal of data aggregation is to connect to these various databases through a set of plug-and-play connectors. Companies such as Talend and DeepDomain offer such connectors while others like Informatica offer the meta-data management functions. The ideal analytics systems should be able to 'crawl' through a healthcare institution's infrastructure and discover data tables and databases residing on different servers. Such a system would locate all Access databases (by file type) or SQL server databases and allow connection to them by ODBC connectors. For a healthcare-specific use-case, consider Figure 1.3 that shows aggregation of data across many modalities and repositories the Data-Bus architecture that was shown in Figure 1.2-B. This single view provides the workflow overlay of front-office and back-office activities that are enhanced and optimized through data analytics.

1.7 Analytics Layer

In this layer, a data scientist uses a number of engines to carry the analytical functions. Depending on the task at hand, a data scientist may use one or multiple engines to build an analytics application. A more complete layer would include engines for optimization, machine learning, natural language processing, predictive modeling, pattern recognition, classification, inferencing and semantic analysis.

Optimization engine is used to optimize and find the best possible solution to a given problem. Optimization engine is used to identify the best combination of other variables to give an optimal result. Optimization is often used to find lowest cost, the highest utilization or optimal level of care among several possible decision options.

Machine learning is a branch of artificial intelligence that is concerned with construction and building of programs that learn from data. This is a basis for building adaptive models and algorithms that learn from data as well as adapt their performance to data as data changes over time or when applied to one population versus another. For example, models based on machine learning can automatically classify patients into groups of having a disease or not-having a disease.

Natural language processing (NLP) is a field of computer science and artificial intelligence that builds computer understanding of spoken language and texts. NLP has many applications, but in the context of analyzing unstructured data, an NLP engine can extract relevant structured data from the structured text. When combined with other engines, the extracted text can be analyzed for a variety of applications. One of the applications is to automatically search and extract quality measures from medical notes or to prepare COAP and registry reports automatically.

Predictive modeling engine provides the algorithms used for making predictions. This engine would include several statistical and mathematical models that data scientists can use to make predictions. An example is making prediction about patient re-admissions after discharge. Typically, these engines ingest historical data and learn from the data to make predictions. In Part II, we'll review some of the techniques for predictive modeling in more detail.

Pattern recognition engines, also known as data mining programs, provide tools for data scientists to discover associations and patterns in data. These tools enable data scientists to identify shape and patterns in data, perform correlation analysis and clustering of data in multiple dimensions. Some of these methods identify outliers and anomalies in data which help data scientists identify black-swan events in their data or identify suspicious or unlikely activity and behavior. Using pattern recognition algorithms, data scientists are able to identify inherent associate rules from the data associations. This is called association rule learning.

Another technique is building a regression model which works to define a mathematical relationship between data variables with minimum error. When the data includes discrete numbers, regression models work fine. But, when data includes a mix of numbers and categorical data (textual labels), then logistic regression is used. There are linear and non-linear regression models and since many data associations in biological systems are inherently non-linear, the more complete engines provide non-linear logistic regression methods in addition to linear models.

Classification engines solve the problem of identifying which set of categories a subject or data element belongs. There are two approaches, a supervised method and unsupervised method. The supervised methods use a historical set of data as the training set where prior category membership is known. The unsupervised methods use the data associations to define classification categories. The unsupervised classification is also referred to as clustering of data. Classification engines help data scientists to group patients, or procedures, physicians and other entities based on their data attributes.

Inference is the process of reasoning using statistics and artificial intelligence methods to draw a conclusion from data sets. Inference engines include tools and algorithms for data scientists to apply artificial intelligence reasoning methods to their data. Often the result of their inferencing analysis is to answer the question "what should be done next?" where a decision is to be made from observations from data sets. Some inference engines use rule-based approaches that mimic an expert person's process of decision making collected into an expert system. Rules can be applied in a forward chain or backward chain process. In a forward chain process, inference engines start with the known facts and assert new facts until a conclusion is reached. In a backward chain process, inference engines start with a goal and work backward to find the facts needed to be asserted so the goal can be achieved.

Semantic analyzers are analytics engines that build structures and extract concepts from a large set of textual documents. These engines do not require prior semantic understanding of the documents. For example, computer-assisted coding (CAC) applications extract concepts from medical notes and apply semantic analysis to determine polarity and meaning of text; if a diagnosis term is positive, negative, speculative, conditional or hypothetical.

Machine Learning: Another form of data processing is machine learning. Machine learning is a discipline outgrowth of Artificial Intelligence. Machine learning methods learn from data patterns and can imitate intelligent decisions, perform complex reasoning and make predictions. Medical Predictive analytics use machine learning techniques to make predictions. These algorithms process data at the same rate as they receive data in real time, but they also have a feed-back loop mechanism. The feedback loop takes the output of the analytics system and uses it as input. By processing and comparing their output to the real world outcome, they can fine-tune their learning algorithms and adapt to new changes in data. In this book, we will explore a framework that considers both feed-back loop and feed-forward mechanisms.

Statistical Analysis: Statistical Analysis tools would include descriptive functions such as min, max, mode, median, plus ability to define distribution curve, scatter plot, z-Test, Percentile calculations, and outlier identification. Additional statistical analysis methods would include Regression (Trending) analysis, correlation, Chi-square, maxima and minima calculations, t-Test and F-test, and other methods. For more advanced tools, one can use an open source tool developed at Stanford called MADLIB, (www.madlib.net). Also, Apache Mahout includes a library of open source data analytics functions. Details of these methods can be found in most statistics text books and is out of scope in this book.

Forecasting & Predictive Analytics: Forecasting and predictive analytics are the new frontiers in medical data analytics. The simplest approach to forecasting is to apply regression analysis to calculate regression line and the parameters of the equation line such as the slope and intercept value. Other forecasting methods use interpolation and extrapolation. Advanced forecasting tools offer other types of analyses such as multiple regression, non-linear regression, Analysis of variance (ANOVA) and Multi-variable Analysis of variance (MANOVA), Mean Square Error (MSE) calculations, and residual calculations. A common technique in medical research is logistic regression. Logistic regression is essentially a regular regression analysis except that the variables in the study can be categorical data.

The values of slope and intercept can be used as indicators equations to make predictions. A variation of this technique allows identification of outliers as we shall see in the future chapters.

Predictive Analytics is intended to provide insight into future events. It is model-driven and includes methods that produce predictions using supervised and unsupervised learning. Some of the methods include neural networks, PCA and Bayesian Network algorithms. Predictions require the user to select the predictive variables and the dependent variables from the prediction screen.

A number of algorithms are available in this category that together provides a rich set of analytics functionality. These algorithms include Logistic Regression, Naive Bayes, Decision trees and Random forest, regression trees, linear and non-linear regression, Time Series ARIMA[11], ARTXp, and Mahout analytics (Collaborative Filtering, Clustering, Categorization). Additional advanced statistical analysis tools are often used, such as multivariate logistic regression, Kalman filtering, Association rules, LASSO and Ridge regression, Conditional Random Fields (CRF) methods, and Cox Proportional Hazard models to support text extractions. A brief mathematical overview of these techniques appears in Chapter 5.

Pattern Analysis: Using machine learning algorithms researchers can detect patterns in data, perform classification of patient population, and cluster data by various attributes. The algorithms used in this analysis include various neural networks methods, Principal Component Analysis (PCA), Support Vector Machines, supervised and unsupervised learning methods such as k-means clustering, logistic regression, decision tree, and support vector machines.

Other methods include graphical reasoning, a form of case-based reasoning. These techniques enable the researcher to identify a specific clinical case and then search through the clinical data and identify other cases that match the specific clinical case. These methods and their statistical algorithms are explained in more detail in Chapter 5.

1.8 Presentation Layer

This layer includes tools for building dashboards, applications and user-facing applications that display the results of analytics engines. Data scientists often mash up several dashboards (called "Mashboards") on the screen to display the results using infographic graphs. These dashboards are active and display data dynamically as the underlying analytics models continuously update the results for dashboards.

Infographic dashboards allow us to visualize data in a more relevant way with better illustrations. These dashboards may combine a variety of charts, graphs and visuals together. Chapter 3 contains a more in-depth

---

[11] Auto Regressive Integrated Moving Average.

coverage of infographic components including heat maps, tree maps, bar graphs, variety of pie charts and parallel charts and many more visualization forms.

Advanced presentation layers include data visualization tools that allows data scientist to easily visualize the results of various analyses (classification, clustering, regression, anomaly detection, etc.) in an interactive and graphical user interface.

Several companies provide rapid data visualization programs including Tableau, QlikView, Panopticon, Pentaho and Logi which are revolutionizing how we view data in healthcare. Panopticon has developed a Complex Event Processor (CEP) engine that allows users to view patient prior events in graphical representations. Soon 3-Dimensional (3D) and Multi-Dimensional (mD) visualization tools will be widely adopted in the healthcare industry providing rich and rapid view into patient data and clinical operations.

The EMR systems architecturally belong to this layer. The challenge with implementing analytics-driven workflows served up by the EMR systems remains to be their "openness" to integration. Those EMR systems that allow tight integration with analytics engines and models will enable the enterprise to achieve analytics-driven workflows more quickly than others.

1.9 Clinical Intelligence process

Clinical Intelligence follows a series of steps, typically along the sequence of the following eight key steps. The First 3 steps are commonly referred to as Extract-Transfer-Load (ETL). The remaining steps explain the data ingestion into analytics platform and processing the data:

1. Data integration (Extraction). Data integration (or data extraction) is possible with EMR systems such as EPIC, Cerner, McKesson, Intergy, Meditech, Siemens Soarian and a number of other EMR systems by simply cloning the existing HL7 interfaces. Data integration with data warehouse systems such as Microsoft Amalga can be performed via SQL Services Integration Services (SSIS) or SQL Services Report Services (SSRS).

2. Data Transformation. Often data needs to be either normalized or transformed across multiple sources to conform to a common standard, such as a common format or common data elements.

3. Data Ingestion (Load). In this step the data is properly ingested by the Clinical Intelligence system and imported into the appropriate data structure. The ingested data can be structured data fields or unstructured text such as physician notes and charting information.

4. Term Extraction. Using Natural Language Processing (NLP) technologies, the ingested data is parsed and pertinent clinical data are extracted from unstructured data.

5. Semantic Analysis. Once the clinical terms are extracted, their relationships, strength and acuity must be established. Semantic analytics provides the intelligent means to identify meaning and relationships between patient and various medical terms.

6. Statistical analysis. Given the frequency and distribution of extracted data, certain statistical inference can be made about the data. Such inferences provide information about outliers, trends, clusters of data and Pareto analysis.

7. Pattern Analysis. Advanced techniques borrowed from Artificial Intelligence techniques such as artificial neural networks, case-based analysis and machine learning algorithms are used to identify patterns, causal relationships, influence diagrams, classification of data and predictive analysis.

8. Meta-Analysis. This stage considers results of all other analytical steps and models to make an overall set of conclusions and insight about the data that has been analyzed.

1.10 Clinical Intelligence Maturity Model

Clinical Intelligence can be viewed from an evolutionary perspective of increasing functionality. The utility of these functions and their benefits are described in a maturity model as shown in Figure 1.4.

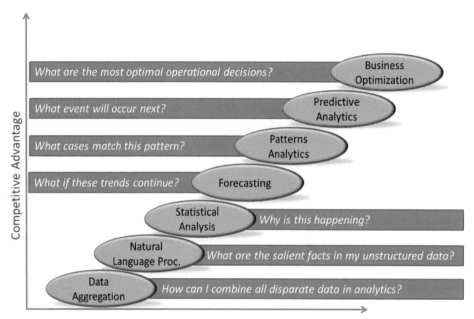

Fig. 1.4- Hierarchy of Analytics Functionality

1.11 Applications of Analytics in Medicine

One regional hospital in Italy uses SAS analytic tools for its analytics to improve a variety of patient-centric workflows and processes. The hospital was able to improve management control over movement and transportation of patients, materials, reports and provisioning of goods and services. By establishing four standards for measurement and analysis the hospital was able to improve bed utilization efficiency, reduced average length of stay (LOS) and overall costs by more than 20%. The four major standard pillars for measurement and analysis consisted of: 1) developing standards for measuring and standardizing patient-care activities, 2) developing metrics and indicators plus monitoring systems to measure such metrics, 3) improved the auditing process to audit for performance, and 4) working to manage risk for patients and staff better.

Clinical Intelligence promises to transform relevant big data into true business value by enabling management to make more informed and insightful decisions. The right analytics tools are scalable and re-usable for future data sets plus they are adaptable to new types of data.

Clinical Intelligence is used to measure and inform care providers of their compliance with care guidelines. For example, before a patient visits a practice, the doctor can be informed of any pre-conditions or required treatment to ensure compliance with care guidelines. Analytics are used to develop health plan management tools and product. One organization used Clinical Intelligence to determine which population of children needed certain immunizations. Such information was helpful to send a notification to those children and administer immunization during patient's visit (SAS 2011)

Clinical Intelligence is not only applied at the enterprise level but also across several institutions and regions covering thousands of doctors and practices. Day-to-day data is collected and benchmarked and analyzed using big data analytics tools. Similarly, the goal of many organizations is to benchmark relative to national norms and population insight to let doctors know what they can anticipate relative to the population.

But even descriptive statistics has not been fully utilized in healthcare. Most institutions are just starting to analyze and understand the impact of variation in their outcomes, costs, reimbursements and care-related activities. Study of variation of practice patterns explains where over-use or under-use of medical care for a given condition and within a particular specialty has occurred.

1.12 Data Mining of Medical Data

An advanced form of Business Intelligence called Data Mining has received tremendous attention and popularity once its competitive value and early success stories were published. Data Mining attempts to find associations and relationships between data elements that are not obvious. Clinical Intelligence uses data mining techniques to identify such relationships and associations between data elements and data sets.

Projects such as Non-Obvious Relationship Awareness (NORA) and Data Mining software probe databases searching for obscure matches and relations between relevant information. This approach can identify connections between data that can span as many as 30 degrees of separation. One degree of separation would be two patients developing the same hospital acquired infection. The second degree would be finding out that both patients visited the same CT scanner room. A third degree might be discovering that the same transporter transferred those patients.

This approach is known as the "Black-box" method where the analyst makes no prior assumptions about the data and inter-relations about the data. There is also a "White-box" approach, where the causal relationships between data are known to the analyst. Clinical Intelligence builds upon all these methods and technologies to overcome the inherent complexity of clinical data analysis extract appropriate and relevant information and then analyze it with both Black-box and White-box methods.

1.13 Clinical and Business Optimization

The goal of Clinical and Business Optimization is to use Clinical Intelligence to navigate through key performance indicators of the organization and identify functions that need further optimization and improvement. At this level, the executive management team can view the entire clinical and business operations through key metrics provided in form of data visualization tools such as Dashboards.

The system allows users to select certain variables such as quality core measures, or balance score card metrics and keep a "watch" on these variables. The user is able to compose a dashboard of variables. The outcome is displayed as a dashboard. The user can drill down on certain variables for more detail or conversely roll-up to the higher level of dashboard display. From the detailed view, the user can select certain variables and perform knowledge discovery and analytics all over again.

At this level of maturity, hospitals use the results of their Clinical Intelligence reports to improve clinical processes, implement Lean workflows, reduce hospital acquired complications (HAC) and gain appropriate reimbursements. Chapter 3 provides sample dashboards including a balanced score card method that captures the four elements of financials, clinical quality, patient satisfaction and business operational measures.

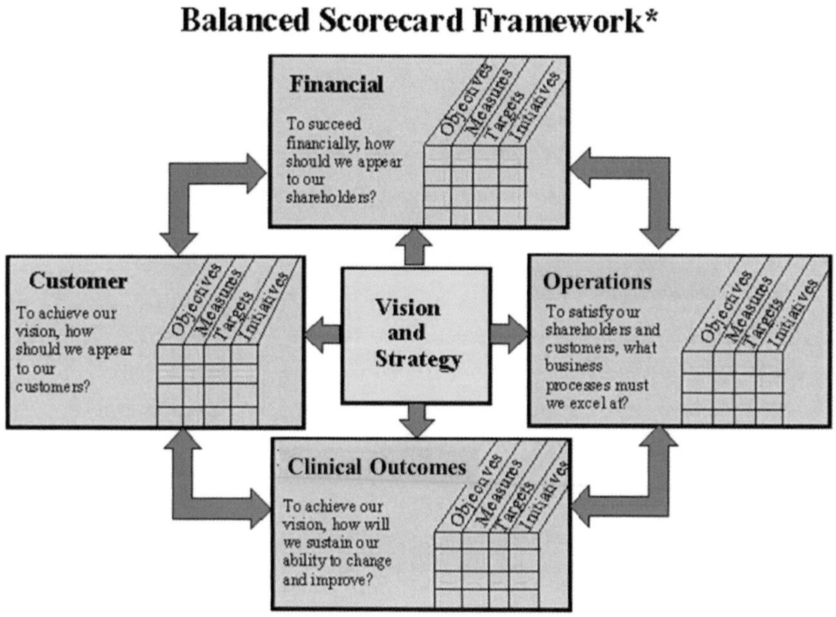

Balanced Scorecard Framework*

* Adapted from Kaplan & Norton 1996. *The Balanced Scorecard*. Harvard Business School Press: 9. Original from HBR Jan/Feb 1996, p. 76.

Fig. 1.5- Balanced Score Card as Driver for Measurements and Analytics

1.14 Key Considerations in Clinical Intelligence Reports

When organizing a Clinical Intelligence report, several factors should be considered. These factors include:

Content: What will you measure?

Audience: Who is your audience?

Production: Who will be responsible for data and distribution?

Accuracy: How will you ensure the accuracy of information?

Frequency: How frequently should the report be distributed?

Format: What is the ideal format for the report?

Usage: How will the information be used?

Accountability: Who is accountable for performance metrics and clinical data reports?

Response: What is the expected and required response to the data presented in the report? What actions are necessary as responses to the report?

1.15 The Elements of a Clinical Intelligence Program

Larger organizations are likely to combine their business intelligence and clinical intelligence plans into a single data analytics program for maximum effectiveness. A typical Clinical and Business Intelligence program contains four pillars as described below (Figure 1.8):

Pillar 1: Data Analytics Strategy

Every Clinical Intelligence Program must define its purpose, goals and objectives and how it intends to support the organizations strategy. There must be a linkage between the organization's strategy and data analytics strategy. The best practice strategies should answer questions such as:

- How do our data analytics plans map to the organization's strategic goals?
- What is our long range plan for data analytics? The ideal time horizon is to consider a 5-year plan and a 10-year plan.
- What are the strategic plans for analytics? What are the priorities for these analytics objectives?
- How does our analytics plan meet the operational, financial and clinical initiatives?
- How will data analytics be transformative in our organization?

Pillar #2: Data Analytics Governance

Data Analytics Governance is concerned with establishing policies and scope of data analytics. Best practices recommend forming a Data Analytics Governance Committee as a sub-committee to the IT organization's Governance board. This pillar is concerned with answering and guiding the following questions:

- What are our standards for data warehousing and data management across the enterprise?
- What are the security, usage policies and privacy guidelines? Who has ownership to what data and do we have their permission to use that data for analytics?
- What are the proper and appropriate applications of analytics? Specify the improper and banned uses of analytics.
- Who will own the results of analytics and the derivative data and models that are developed from our data? Who will own the intellectual property of the results that we'll discover through analytics?

Pillar #3: Data Analytics Framework

The Framework deals with technical aspects of managing data and analytics tools. It answers questions about:

- What are the infrastructure requirements today and in 5-10 years? Should we build an on premise cloud infrastructure or store data in an off premise private virtual cloud? What are the infrastructure components for data storage and archiving?
- Which systems of record will be supported and designated as analytics platforms? The answer typically starts with existing data warehouse assets and vendor commitments. For example, a hospital system that has invested in EPIC Clarity, Cognos and SAS is likely to elect these components as a starting point as its systems of record for analytics.
- What analytics tools will we support and what will our analytics tools library consist of?
- What technologies and vendor solutions will be supported as enterprise analytics systems to provide infrastructure and analytics tools?
- What is our analytics capability roadmap? What solutions do we intend to deploy in the next 5 years and in what priority?

Pillar #4: Data Analytics Community

This pillar is concerned with the community of users, meeting their expectations and user's perspective. Questions that the analytics program must address include:

- What are the use-cases and analytics needs plus areas of opportunity for applying analytics?
- Who is the typical user and the user persona for analytics? Note that there are several personas in a large organization that ranges from financial manager to clinical Quality manager, from physician researcher to the C-suite CMO's office. In a large organization as many as a dozen personas are typical.
- Who produces analytics dashboards (or reports) and who will consume them?
- What are the standards for internal publishing and subscribing to analytics results? The people who produce dashboards and perform the analytics work are typically data scientists and data analysts. In a publish-and-subscribe model, the analysts are publishing their dashboards and the users subscribe (or consume) those reports.
- What is the expected usage model from user community? This can define the Service Level Agreement (SLA) between the users and the data analytics group at your organization. The Data Analytics Program should define the role of the user with respect to analytics. Do we provide a self-service model or a DIY (Do-IT-Yourself) model where we provide the infrastructure and analytics tools so the users perform their own analytics and develop their own applications? In contrast, do we provide a full-service concierge desk similar to Data Marts so that the IT organization performs the analytics and users can consume analytics as-a-services (AaaS).

Analytics Strategy	Analytics Governance	Analytics Framework	Analytics Community
Strategic Plan Perspective	**Policy Management Perspective**	**Infrastructure Perspective**	**User Community Perspective**
How data analytics plans map to organizational goals?	What are the standards for data warehousing & data management?	What infrastructure components are in scope?	What are the use-cases and who are the users?
What is our long range (5-10 year) plan for analytics?	What are the security, privacy, ownership rights & usage policies for analytics?	What are the systems of record for analytics?	Who produces analytics dashboards and who consumes them?
What are the strategic plans for analytics?	What are the guidelines for proper application of analytics?	What will the standard tools library consist of?	What are the standards for internal publishing and subscription of analytic results?
How does analytics meet the operational, financial and clinical initiatives?	Who will own the derivative analytics data and intellectual property?	What technologies will be supported for infrastructure, analytics and visualization?	Usage methods: self-service or concierge?
How will analytics be transformative?		What is our analytics capability roadmap?	Community of analytics users (publishers & subscribers)

Fig. 1.6 – The Four Pillars of Data Analytics Program

Overall the key questions and decisions regarding data management that are needed to be made include five areas:

- What is our data model going to be?
- What is the query model?
- What is our data consistency model?
- What applications and APIs are required to meet our business strategy and analytics needs?
- What is the data analytics user community and how to involve them into the decision making process?

A best practice in data analytics program suggests that we take inventory of data and map them against the organization's analytics needs. A tool for capturing a high level map is using the Data Analytics Matrix. Figure 1.7 illustrates a typical Data Analytics Matrix which includes the analytics requirements in the column heading and the rows below it define: the purpose, priority, user community, required data, sources of data, available data warehouses, any data access limitations, data types, data quality, analytics methods required and user interface for each column.

Analytics use case vs. Governance Criteria	Readmission Prediction	Revenue Cycle Leakage Analysis	Clinical Quality Metrics	Population Health Management	Clinical-Translational Medicine Research	Genomics-Precision Medicine Research
Purpose	Predict readmission	Increase revenue capture	Quality reports	Manage population health	Evidence-based medicine	Clinical discovery & advancement
Priority	Med	Hi	Hi	Lo	Med	Hi
User Community	Discharge Nurse	CFO office	Quality & Compliance Office	Primary Care Physician community	Specialists, Clinicians	Life Science researchers
Required Data	Medical billing codes	Medical billing codes + medical records	Medical records	Medical records	Medical records	Genomics data + medical records
Data Source(s)	Billing Systems	Billing system + EMR	EMR	EMR + Billing system	EMR	EMR + Genetic sequence data
Data Warehouse	No	No	Yes	Yes	No	Yes
Data Access Issues	ETL possible	ETL possible	Limited	Limited	HL7 extract possible	ETL possible
Data Type (Structured / Unstructured?)	Structured	Structured	Structured + unstructured	Structured + unstructured	Structured + unstructured	Structured + unstructured
Data Quality	Excellent	Excellent	Good	Average	Average	Good
Analytics methods	Predictive modeling	Rule-based method	Descriptive Statistics	Classification methods	Logistic regression	Bayes Nets, Neural Networks
User interface	Workflow driven dashboards	Audit dashboards	Dashboards with drill-down feature	Dashboards with drill-down feature	Dashboard with drill-down feature	Dashboard with link to medical records

Fig. 1.7 – Example of a Data Analytics Matrix

1.16 The Seven Axioms of Big Data Analytics:

So far, we've covered a vast area about big data, analytics and potential use cases of applying analytics to clinical data. In this final section Chapter 1, I'd like to share some general observations that I've collected as axioms about Big Data Analytics.

Mathematics has become Biology's new microscope and the new telescope for astronomy. The vast amount of data being generated in biology, physical sciences and business are providing the enormous empirical evidence leading scientists and managers to use mathematical sciences as the new microscope or telescopes for discovery in their field. Just as astronomers in the 17th century spent most of their times on building telescopes and less time viewing stars, today's data scientists are spending much of their time building models. But, that will change as standard analytics platforms will emerge to handle Big Data volumes. Analytics platforms that provide the standard data "scope" will be widely adopted.

1. **More data is better.** The more data is available, the richer the insight and results that big data analytics can produce. Unlike descriptive statistics which is less interested in outliers and more on the central tendency of data frequency, in Big Data Analytics, outliers and black swan events are of more interest. Our ability to produce knowledge from Big Data is only limited by our capacity to store and process that data. The bigger and more diverse the data set, the better the analysis can model the real-world. Try to incorporate as many data sets from internal and public sources as possible.

2. **One model does not fit ALL.** Most scientists and data analysts work hard to find the best model or algorithm that meets their data challenges. But, that approach will fail the challenges for a scalable and extensible that result from the dynamic nature of real world data. As the saying goes, one size does not fit all, a single algorithm does not meet diversity of data sets and changes in data that may occur over time. Hence, as I proposed in my doctoral dissertation, the data scientist must build a committee of models that collectively can produce a more intelligent, adaptable and scalable analytics solution immune to variants of data.

3. **BI and analytics are not the same things.** Where Business intelligence (BI) comes short, Big Data Analytics thrives. When we run business intelligence reports, we're extracting data that are structured, normalized, limited in scope, often relational and well behaved. The business intelligence techniques fail when we deal with very large and diverse amount of data, unstructured data that's typically found in textual files, noisy or missing data and data that is not in tabular format. While BI is concerned with descriptive statistics and simple mathematical manipulations of structured data, Big Data Analytics comes with tools such as Natural Language Processing (NLP) to extract data from unstructured text, or with pattern recognition models, predictive models, optimization and machine learning. BI has the power to show snapshots of data presented in graphs. In contrast, Big Data Analytics provides analysis of data through real-time data analysis with feedback that improves the models over time and the results are provided through data visualization tools.

4. **Correlation and causality are not the same.** While positive or negative correlations tell us a lot about relationships between data elements and variables, they don't constitute causality. It takes a lot more to claim one variable is the cause for another. For example, we must show that one variable occurs in time before the other. And, that the spurious variable effects –the indirect effect of other variables- are properly accounted for. But, this is not to discourage seeking the root cause of events, it's to emphasize that interpretive skills are just as important as mathematical modeling talents. Data

scientists should have the interpretive skills that go beyond the mathematical abilities to interpret the results of analysis. What do all these correlations tell us and what changes can produce the desired outcomes.

5. **Sparse data analytics approaches will win.** As the volume of data increases, the likelihood that data sets will contain noisy, duplicated data or the opposite, miss important data elements will increase. Hence, whenever we collect massive amount of data, we should anticipate and prepare to cleanse data, de-duplicate and handle sparse data sets. The sparseness will naturally increase as the data volumes rise over time. Therefore, the sparse data analytics methods will eventually overshadow the dense data analytics methods.

6. **Machine learning and Data mining are not the same, but cousins.** Machine learning is a branch of artificial intelligence that provides systems that can learn from data. Machine learning is often used to classify data or make predictions, based on known properties in the data learned from historical data that's used for training. Data mining works to provide insights and discovery of unknown properties in the data.

   Machine learning can be done by supervised learning or unsupervised learning methods. The unsupervised learning uses algorithms that operate on unlabeled data, namely, the data input where the desired output is unknown. The goal is to discover structure in the data but not to generalize a mapping between inputs to outputs. The supervised learning use labeled data for training. Labeled data are datasets where the input and outputs are known. The supervised learning method work to generalize a relationship or mapping between inputs to outputs. There is an overlap between the two. Often data mining uses machine learning methods and vice versa, where machine learning can use data mining techniques, such as unsupervised learning to improve the engine training more accurate.

7. **Use Signal boosting methods.** When data is sparse and the number of data variables grows large, we face a multi-dimensionality challenge. We rely on signal boosting methods to overcome multi-dimensionality issue to improve model accuracy and performance. Signal boosting increases the significance of certain data variables (which otherwise would have small significance) in data mining and predictive modeling such that their contributions are weighted higher.

1.17 Natural Language Processing

Much of Big Data in healthcare is in unstructured format. More than 80% of the data is in form of narrative text and notes, not in discrete data fields. It would be a major advantage to have a natural language processing (NLP) tool integrated into the analytics process. The ideal NLP tool not only extracts data but also presents the extraction along with relationships to other data to create an interim structured dataset which can be used for further processing.

The ideal NLP tool is equipped with some semantic processing capability. Simple semantic processing functions would include synonyms, identify associations as defined by user, exclusions (such as exclude all negative cases or certain phrases) and provide simple frequency count of phrase occurrence.

Advanced Semantic processing will support meaning extraction by clustering phrases, creating graphs of sentence structures. Semantic processors map these structures to concepts in the UMLS domain model. The user will be able to define the variants of a noun. For example to define variants of the phrase Ocular

Complications, the user (or the tool might suggest) entering synonyms and variants such as: ocular, oculars, oculus, oculi, eyepiece, ophthalmic, ophthalmia, optic, optics, complication, complications, and so on.

As another example, when a user searches for "Use of thermogram in detection of meningitis", the semantic feature of the tool would identify Meningitis as a disease and thermogram as a method. Notice a representative semantic sentence structure built by a semantic analyzer that might look like a structure in Figure 1.8. These internal structures maintain relationships and meaning that are key to intelligent term extraction from medical records.

Semantic Analysis: "Use of Thermogram in Detection of Meningitis"

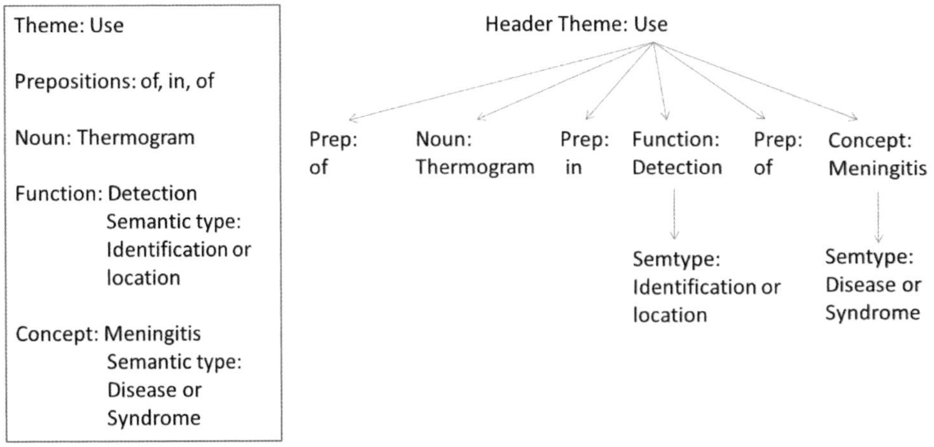

Fig. 1.8. Example of Possible Semantic Analysis of a Search Phrase

For general data exploration, the system can use MeSH[12] hierarchy or UMLS to create different categories. Other categories can be supplied by the researcher. The top-level categories in the MeSH descriptor hierarchy are:

MeSH Hierarchy	
Anatomy [A]	Anthropology, Education, Sociology and Social Phenomena [I]
Organisms [B]	Technology and Food and Beverages [J]
Diseases [C]	Humanities [K]
Chemicals and Drugs [D]	Information Science [L]
Analytical, Diagnostic and Therapeutic Techniques and Equipment [E]	Persons [M]
Psychiatry and Psychology [F]	Health Care [N]
Biological Sciences [G]	Publication Characteristics [V]
Physical Sciences [H]	Geographic Locations [Z]

---

[12] Medical Subject Heading (MeSH) and Unified Medical Language System (UMLS)

The references to meningitis and thermogram can be clustered by classes of documents or other subjects to produce a more refined search result. Certain search results can be presented using 3-Dimenstional data visualization tools.

The researcher is able to manipulate this representation by rotating in 3D space. Additional functions are typically offered to allow researcher to expand or clip and bound certain edges and then select certain extracted terms to perform additional semantic analytics. The thickness of each line can represent the strength of relationship between the topics. This data visualization technique offers new opportunities for data exploration among unstructured data.

Chapter 2. Clinical Intelligence Use Cases

Clinical Intelligence applications and use cases are found in every aspect of healthcare and medical decision making. Care providers need tools such as clinical decision support applications to order appropriate exams and tests. Insurance companies are increasingly requiring Clinical decision support and evidence based medicine practices including pay for performance to physicians and hospitals. There are common questions that hospital administrators, physicians and care quality managers want to answer.

2.1 Use Cases

In order to illustrate clinical intelligence applications and what clinical intelligence can offer, several clinical intelligence use cases are described here.

- Inpatient Length of Stay Management – Reduce the patient length of stay so hospital capacity can increase. Use statistical methods to identify the patient cases that can be discharged sooner.
- At Risk Population Detection – Identify which population of patients are risk of diseases that can be prevented, such as patients missing required vaccinations.
- Readmissions Management – Ensure that patients discharged don't return within 30-90 days after discharge.
- Chronic Disease Detection - Identify which patients have early markers for chronic diseases such as diabetes, hypertension, etc.
- Hospital Acquired Condition Prevention – Identify and predict hospital acquired infections and complications such as Pulmonary Embolism and Deep Vein Thrombosis.
- Chronic Care Management – Track treatments and prevention plans for patients with chronic diseases.
- Tailored Benefit Design – identify opportunities for packaging care plans for ACO and insurance companies using data analytics that define the cost basis and margin across a population of patients.
- Additional use cases are described at the end of this chapter.

2.2 Clinical Risk Stratification

The goal of risk stratification is to properly and accurately classify patient's health condition in the appropriate risk level. This has at least two important ramifications: First, physicians are able to make more informed and justified clinical care decisions and second, the proper DRG payment levels can be assigned to such patient care scenarios. Some common Risk stratification use cases can be expressed in terms of clinical quality questions, such as:

- Which patients are likely to return as emergency patients?
- Who is likely to be re-admitted in the next 12 months?
- Which patients are likely to exhibit reaction, Post-Operative Nausea and Vomiting (PONV) to anesthesia?
- Which patients are missing their antibiotic or other medication at the current time?
- Hospital administrators want to know which patients should receive a special medication, treatment or intervention. For example, which patients should receive H1N1 or TB vaccine?
- Which patients are missing their antibiotics post-surgery?
- Which patients are receiving a medication that they are allergic to?

- Are there patients in the hospital who have received medications that have drug-drug or drug-allergy adverse interaction?

The immediate opportunity in clinical intelligence is in diagnosis and clinical decision support today. But the more rewarding opportunity is in medical prediction[13]. The goal of prediction is to predict adverse patient events and medical complications in advance in order to allow adequate time of intervention and prevention. For example, which patients are likely to pose post-surgery reaction to anesthesia? What are the morbidity risks or risks of developing a complication like Deep Vein Thrombosis?

A number of clinical metrics can be tracked over time to provide core quality measures (CQM). These measurements provide the basis for further statistical analysis, dashboards and alerts. In addition to these clinical measures, a user can identify and mark other data variables to include them in their analytics.

2.3 Core & Composite Clinical Measures

An advantage of clinical Intelligence is to offer real-time monitoring and tracking of vital patient care and safety measures. These metrics and measures can be extracted and analyzed routinely. A Composite safety index can be derived from a set of measurements. In addition once a threshold or target value for normal range is set, any value that falls outside of the interval can be set to signal clinical alerts. Some of these measurements are offered below as routinely monitored core measures:

- Bloodstream infections up?
- Respiratory failure rate?
- Pulmonary Embolism trending up?
- UTI[14] down at target vs. last year?
- Diabetics with A1c under control?
- Patients with LDL under control?
- Smokers offered smoking cessation?
- Patients requiring vaccination?

For these measurements, hospital administrators and medical officers expect clinical intelligence analysts to report actual value versus target. They track percent (%) increase, variance from target, and whether the trend is up or down.

2.4 Patient Safety Indicators

There are a number of patient safety indicators that are typically measured and tracked. These indicators are now de-facto standard at most healthcare institutions. Among them are the following Indicators:

- Patients with dehiscence post-surgery
- Patients developing UTI during hospital stay
- Patients with respiratory failure post operatively
- Patients with post-op sepsis

---

[13] "Experiments with Neural Networks as Tools for Medical prognostics", Peter Ghavami & Kailash Kapur, 2011
[14] UTI: Urinary Tract Infection; A1c: A test that gives physicians an idea of how high a patient's glucose levels have been in the last 3 months. A level over 8% is regarded as high; LDL: Low Density Lipoprotein, regarded as the "bad" cholesterol measure.

- Patients with postoperative physiologic and metabolic derangement
- Patients with post op hip fracture
- Patients with fall incidence
- Patients post-op Deep Vein Thrombosis/Pulmonary Embolism (DVT/PE)
- Patients developing decubitus ulcer during hospital stay
- Patients with central venous catheter-related bloodstream infections
- LOS: Observed to expected
- Direct Cost: Observed to Expected
- Mortality: Observed to Expected Ratio
- AHRQ[15] Comorbidity Fluid/Electrolyte
- AHRQ Comorbidity Coagulopathy
- AHRQ Comorbidity Obesity
- AHRQ Comorbidity Weight Loss/Malnutrition
- AHRQ Comorbidity Deficiency Anemia
- AHRQ Comorbidity Heart Failure
- AHRQ Comorbidity Renal failure
- AHRQ Comorbidity Chronic Pulmonary Disease
- Present on Admission - Shock
- Present on Admission - Sepsis
- Present on Admission – Liver Disease
- Present on Admission – Renal Disease

2.5 Clinical Operations Excellence

In addition to the measurements mentioned above, there other categories of clinical operations excellence that are monitored. All of these measurements provide a rich dataset that can be analyzed further with statistical tools to bring additional insight to the clinical decision maker.

- STEMI (ST Elevation Myocardial Infarction) - A number of measures related to patient "Door to balloon" time in Emergency Department.
- OR first surgery start time
- Average Patient wait time in ER before seen by a doctor
- Number of Hospital Acquired Complications (HAC) by type of complication, by service line and by patient demographics
- Trend lines and measurements of data elements that represent the root cause analysis of these factors above over time

2.6 Balanced Score Card: Operational & Quality Dashboards

Dashboards are a form of reports that are typically highly graphical and can show as many as Key Performance Indicator (KPIs) or metrics on a single screen. Common Dashboard analytics can be devised around

---

[15] AHRQ: Agency for Healthcare Research & Quality, a federal agency charged with improving healthcare quality, safety, efficiency and effectiveness of care.

a Balanced Score card. One such representative dashboard includes Financial, Operational, clinical outcome and patient satisfaction measures. These dashboards include metrics, their target values and actual measured performance. The performance is color coded as green, yellow or red to indicate whether the measured metric meets the target value.

Most dashboards allow drill-down and roll-up functions. Drill-down give the user the ability to quickly navigate through highly summarized data to see the underlying detailed data. It can help the users to understand cause-and-effect relationships. A roll-up function allows users to start from detailed data view to the more aggregate summaries and eventually to the single dashboard view. A sample list of measurements for Balanced Score Card report may include the following values:

Financial Measures:
- Hospital (Tot Inc / Tot Oper Rev) - (Budg Tot Inc / Budg Tot Oper Rev)
- Hospital Ambulatory Specialty Clinic Visits
- Hospital IP + OP (inpatient and outpatient) Operating Room (OR) Volumes
- Hospital Admissions
- Hospital Case Mix Index
- Hospital ED Visits
- Hospital FTEs
- Hospital Payer Mix Commercial
- Hospital Payer Mix Unsponsored
- FYTD Mean LOS (All units)

Operational Measures:
- Hospital Patient Days - Budget Variance
- Hospital Mean LOS - Budget Variance
- Hospital Occupancy Rate - Budget Variance
- OP First OR Starts (within 5mins)
- IPA OR First Starts (within 5mins)
- Increase Referrals to specialty care (w/ appts)
- ED % Left without being seen
- Concurrence with Transfer Criteria
- Mental Health Integration (contacts)

Clinical Outcome Measures:
- Hospital Patient Days - Budget Variance
- Hospital Mean LOS - Budget Variance
- Hospital Occupancy Rate - Budget Variance
- Nosocomial MRSA Rate
- Central Line-Associated Bloodstream Infection Rate
- Hand Hygiene Compliance - Inpatient (IP) and outpatient (OP)
- Harm Events (compared to national average or ranking reported by UHC and AHRQ)
- Mortality: Observed to Expected Ratio

- Core Measures Aggregate Score
- Diabetic Ambulatory Weighted Average
- Cancer Screening Weighted Average
- Median Time to Fibrinolysis
- Fibrinolytic Therapy with in 30min of ED Arrival
- Median time to transfer to another facility for Acute Coronary Care
- Aspirin at Arrival
- Median time to ECG
- Timing of Antibiotic Prophylaxis
- Prophylactic Antibiotic selection for surgery patients

Patient Satisfaction:
- Inpatient Patience Experience – HCAHPS Overall Patient Rating
- Hospital Employee Turnover YTD

For all these measures, clinical data analyst is expected to provide actual values versus budgeted (or target) values, percent (%) variance, and trend line to indicate whether the trend data is moving up or down.

2.7 Clinical Intelligence for Safety and Risk Management

With the Clinical Intelligence approach, you can quickly and easily find the patient populations that may (or may not) be meeting key Quality criterion. Clinical Intelligence allows users to easily identify patients that met, or failed to meet Quality criteria.

How quickly do you want to identify every document that mentions Heparin, Arixta or Fragmin in the last 30 days? Or in the last 90 days? or the last Year? As routine function of Clinical Intelligence, the clinical data analyst can reconcile the Pharmacy and ADT data for a quality report, then triangulate the distribution of anticoagulants with the documentation for each patient.

Some of the practical aspects of Clinical Intelligence provide the following functions for all users in a hospital environment:

- Determine if patients have a potential drug-drug Interaction issue. This is a Quality Metric that measure Drug-Drug Interaction (DDI)
- Quickly identify potential HF/AMI/Pneumonia, Hip/Knee replacement/COPD or other common ailments 30-day or 90-day re-admissions
- Identify patients who are likely to develop certain hospital acquired complications
- Review 'Aspirin on Arrival' and/or 'Aspirin at Discharge'
- Send an alert each time a patient is admitted that warrants a review by a Quality staff when certain clinical values are present on admission
- Locate every patient that is on Percocet with 3 or more known risk factors
- Locate patients that are on a Nexium dosage of 40mg* or higher with known alcoholism/alcohol abuse & presenting with documented adverse reactions. This is an example of drug over-dose identification when the manufacturer's recommended dose is exceeded. In this scenario, the recommended Nexium dose by the manufacturer is for 20mg.

- Locate patients who were admitted with Cardiac Heart Failure (CHF), AMI, Pneumonia and stroke today or yesterday.
- Identify patients who have a key Core Measures condition so you can disburse appropriate targeted care

2.8 Clinical Documentation Improvement Measures[16]

University Health Consortium maintains a list of performance measures for its member hospitals. Physician queries are regarded as backbone of improving clinical documentation. Query is the process of asking physicians for further explanation about their documentation. The ideal process to query physicians is moving away from retrospectively to concurrent review process. The CDI measures adopted by UHC include:

- CMI, ROM, and SOI values and trends by service and provider
- Percentage of extreme SOI and ROM cases
- Trends in O/E values (mortality, length of stay, and UHC benchmarks)
- Trends in diagnoses and MS-DRGs by service line
- CC/MCC capture rates
- Query response rates by service and provider
- Most common reason for queries
- Percentage of charts queried and not queried
- Percentage of unknown POA diagnoses
- Trends in documentation chart audits
- Internal CDI dashboards: CDS productivity, CDS teaching hours, CDI operating costs, return on investment for severity and financial impact.

2.9 Clinical Intelligence for Clinical Documentation Improvement

With the advent of ICD10 coding regulation more attention is being paid to quality and completeness of Clinical Documentation. Clinical Documentation Improvement (CDI) is rapidly becoming a key area of focus for healthcare facilities. CDI is critical to optimal reimbursement and quality of care. Consider this with the RAC[17] audits where auditors are recovering millions of dollars of reimbursement from poorly documented and/or inappropriately billed encounters. A branch of Clinical Intelligence works to improve CDI. Its goal is to enable CDI staff to efficiently review cases, prioritize and manage their case-load and achieve appropriate reimbursement. Such tools identify patients that may have been 'under' or 'over' documented.

Basic examples of possible 'under' documentation are:

- Cardiac Heat Failure (CHF) Unspecified
    - Find all CHF patients where the clinician failed to mention Systolic *OR* Diastolic,
    - Find all CHF patients where the clinician failed to mention Acute, Chronic *OR* Acute on Chronic
- Diabetic Ketoacidosis (DKA) Unspecified
    - Find all diabetic patients with glucose >250 AND has at least one other valid Lab indicator (pH < 7.3, Anion Gap > 10 *OR* BiCarb < 18) *AND* signs & symptoms that are consistent with Mild DKA

---

[16] POA: Present on Arrival; CDI: Clinical Documentation Improvement; CC/MCC: Comobordity, Complication/Major CC; CDS: ROM: Risk of Mortality; SOI: Severity of Illness;

[17] The Recovery Audit Contractor (RAC) is a program created through the Medicare Modernization Act of 2003 to identify and recover improper Medicare payments to healthcare providers.

- Acute Respiratory Failure Undocumented
  - Find all patients with a Chief Complaint of Shortness of Breath AND PCO2 >50 & pH OR a PO2
- Acute Blood Loss Anemia Undocumented
  - Find all males patients with hemoglobin <13.5 *OR* hematocrit <40, *AND* female patients with a hemoglobin <12 *OR* hematocrit <36 *AND* the diagnosis did not contain "anemia" *AND* the report contains "transfusion"
- When certain disease is mentioned (such as Pneumonia), ask what type or stage of Pneumonia was diagnosed? The physician neglected to state the necessary severity or specificity.
- Missing Signs and symptoms
- Missing Technique
- Missing physician Presence statement
- Missing findings for body area
- Missing Lab tests or results of lab tests
- Route of drug administration (oral, IV or other)not documented
- When the medical record included clinical indicators of a diagnosis, but the physician did not document the condition specifically
- When a physician documented a treatment but not a diagnosis
- When cause-and-effect relationship between two conditions was unclear in the documentation
- When the physician neglected to state the underlying cause of the patient's documented symptoms
- Inconsistencies existed in the documentation of different physicians

CMS has released several guidelines and suggestions on how to prepare for documentation changes and improvements with ICD-10 (CMS 2012)[18]. The ICD-10-CM/PCS code set will require an increased granularity and specificity in documentation as it incorporates laterality, acuity, anatomical specificity and additional combination and complication codes. There are several steps to help facilities begin to parse their documentation and data improvement needs. The Association for Clinical Documentation Improvement Specialists (ACDIS) lists a number of steps to prepare for ICD-10 under-documentation, Including[19]:

- Review systems that use ICD-9 to identify areas in your revenue cycle, reimbursement rates, HIM, electronic medical records, and clinical systems that will eventually use ICD-10.
- Evaluate any potential gaps in clinical conditions or work flow processes that could be affected by increased documentation. Then, update and modify your systems and processes prior to transitioning to the new code sets. This will save your organization time by finding incomplete or non-specific data and ensuring that they do not cause a delay with coding and billing when you finalize implementing ICD-10.
- Evaluate current software systems to determine if existing elements are cost-effective and efficient. If they are not, upgrade, centralize, or replace them before ICD-10 implementation.
- Identify staff members to train right away. Determine who will most benefit from ICD-10 training and how your facility will roll out training to CDI professionals, providers, and coders. Staff who will be using ICD-10

---

[18] Center for Medicare and Medicaid Services, "How to Prepare for Documentation Changes and Improvements with ICD-10", November 2012, http://www.cms.gov/Medicare/Coding/ICD10/index.html?redirect=/ICD10
[19] "Tip: Take Advantage of CMS Tips for ICD-10 Prep", ACDIS, Nov, 21, 2012, http://www.hcpro.com/acdis/details.cfm?topic=WS_ACD_STG&content_id=286636

will need training to become familiar with the increased documentation standards necessary with the new code sets. Training will help staff members become comfortable with both the heightened specificity and increased number of code sets that they will be using frequently.

- Test each stage of the new documentation process in a trial setting. Staff members should simulate a typical patient encounter in its entirety to ensure that data is being documented thoroughly and consistently. This will also help identify any areas that still require improvement in the coding process.

The transition from ICD-9 to ICD-10 offers tremendous challenges that can be resolved with the help of Clinical Intelligence techniques. Some of the metrics, measurements and reports related to ICD-10 transition that a Clinical Intelligence systems can provide is discussed below:

2.10 Current Coding & Billing Key Indicators - Benchmarks

- Current ICD-9 coding analysis and metrics. Provide a baseline analysis of the existing and historical ICD-9 coding practices. This includes key metrics such as:
  - Medicare Case Mix Index (CMI)[20],
  - CC/MCC Capture rate,
  - Unspecified Code usage over a given time period with the ability to drill down into specialty,
  - service line,
  - physician (both attending and operating roles) plus
  - associated DRG/diagnosis codes and
  - CPT/Diagnosis codes.
- Analytical tools can report on both Hospital Billing (HB) and Physician Billing (PB) on key metrics such as:
  - increases/decreases in reimbursements,
  - trends,
  - frequency and Pareto analysis on payments by specialty, physician, patient demographics and payer class.
- The user can set thresholds and automatic alerts to be notified when certain values exceed or go below the threshold.
- Current ICD-9 coding benchmarks. Ability to perform comparisons with national databases such as MedPar[21] and benchmarking across multiple hospital operations.
- Using CMI, the average cost per patient (or by patient day) can be computed relative to the adjusted average cost for other hospitals by dividing the average cost per patient (or patient day) by the hospital's calculated CMI. The adjusted average cost per patient is an indicator of the charges reported for the types of cases treated by that hospital in that year. When a hospital has a CMI of less than 1.00, its adjusted cost per patient will be higher. If a hospital's CMI is greater than 1.00, then the hospital's adjusted cost per patient will be lower.

---

[20] CMI is the average diagnosis-related group (DRG) weight for all of a hospital's Medicare volume.

[21] CMS collects and releases data on all U.S. hospital inpatient stays for Medicare beneficiaries. These data are published by CMS annually under the CMS Medicare Provider Analysis and Review (MedPar) file. The file can be downloaded from http://www.cms.gov/Medicare/Medicare-Fee-for-Service-Payment/AcuteInpatientPPS/FY-2011-IPPS-Final-Rule-Home-Page-Items/CMS1237932.html

- When CMI benchmark data are reported, average Case Mix Index, standard deviation and trending can be provided. Detailed benchmark CMI data can be generated and grouped by specialty, service line and physician based on data from different medical centers for comparison. The data can be collected and ingested from various billing systems (including both Hospital Billing HB and Physician Billing PB) from EPIC, McKesson STAR, GE or other billing systems.
- The benchmarking process allows user to select peer hospitals for comparison based on metrics such as:
  - bed size,
  - geographic location,
  - academic medical center status and Trauma Level
- Additional metrics for benchmarking include:
  - patient age group,
  - sex and race,
  - length of stay (LOS),
  - various categories of accommodation charges,
  - various diagnosis (ICD-9-CM) codes,
  - surgical procedure codes,
  - charges and payment data.
- Financial benchmarks. Analytical tools that compare one hospital with peers in state or across the U.S. are available that provide metrics such as:
  - Total Asset Turnover,
  - Man-hours per discharge,
  - Wage index,
- Benchmarks about hospital market share analysis using state-wide and national data can be provided using Clinical Intelligence tools.

2.11 ICD-9 to ICD-10 Reimbursement Impact

- Inpatient Stay and Discharge data Patterns. Clinical Intelligence tools can discern and detect patterns in data including patient stay and discharge information. Among the patterns and metrics that Clinical Intelligence tools can provide are:
  - Average inpatient length of stay by service line and specialty;
  - discharge status patterns;
  - historical discharge,
  - procedure and diagnosis trends;
  - Patient demographic analysis by state or provider and by peer medical centers selected by user;
  - Average charges,
  - patient diagnosis, and
  - procedure codes by state or by peer medical centers selected by user;
  - Service mix analysis using diagnosis and procedure codes.
- Financial impact of the switch from ICD-9 to ICD-10. Generate reports on potential reimbursement change based on claims analysis and simulated ICD-10 MS-DRGs by specialty, by physician and by patient demographics. Additional metrics can be provided including drill-down into potential reimbursement

impact by individual MS-DRG[22], and by MS-DRG group, by financial class and by payer, plus correlations with patient LOS and other mechanisms such as AP-DRG, APS-DRG, APR-DRG and EAPG[23].

- Impact analysis for certain coding mechanisms. Since Medicare APCs exclude certain outpatient services, EAPG groupings have been adopted by many states. Unlike MS-DRGs, multiple EAPG codes can be applied to the same patient. EAPG provides new opportunities for analytics since it is a visit-based patient classification system directing payment to the main significant procedure or treatment during a visit instead of "a la carte" volume-based purchasing. EAPG data requirements include:
  - Primary diagnosis code,
  - revenue codes,
  - HCPCS codes,
  - Line item dates of service,
  - From/through dates,
  - Condition codes,
  - Age, Gender and
  - Charges
- Certain discounting may apply when different coding systems (MS-DRG vs. APC-DRG vs. EAPG) are used that can be measured using Clinical Intelligence tools. For example, EAPG may apply procedure discounting that modifies reimbursement for an additional procedure provided during the same visit, when multiple significant procedures are performed during the same visit or on the same day and discounts that may apply when bilateral procedures are performed during the same visit or on the same day.
- Managed care contracts. Generate analytical reports of profitability impact on margins related to managed care contracts due to transition to ICD-10.

2.12 Drill-Down Capability and Summary Reports by Coding System

- Financial impact based on specific metrics. Analyze and report medical claims data against medical records to identify financial change due to transition to ICD-10 based on specific ICD-10 diagnosis or CPT codes, plus any triggers for change such as CC/MCC[24] changes, minor procedure switch to becoming a major procedure, changes to principal diagnosis. Reports can provide drill down information to specific service line, specialty, by coder and by physician.
- Coder/CDI specialist understanding of anatomy & physiology. Identify gaps with knowledge and understanding of coders or CDI staff of medical anatomy and physiology by analyzing medical reports against proper ICD-10 coding.
- Coder competency to assign ICD-10-CM and PCS codes. Define and score the coder proficiency in coding to ICD-10-CM and ICD-10-PCS level.

---

[22] DRG: Diagnosis-Related Group. DRGs are used by CMS and other payers to classify diagnosis and procedures that can standardize payments for healthcare services. In 2007, with version 25, CMS introduced MS-DRG with 999 different groups
[23] LOS: Length of Stay, AP-DRG: All Patient DRGs; APR-DRG: All Patient Refined DRGs; APS-DRG: All Patient, Severity-Adjusted DRGs; EAPG: Enhanced Ambulatory Procedure Grouping.
[24] CMS with version 25 of MS-DRG introduced three levels of complications or comorbidities (CC): Absence of CCs, the presence of CCs and a higher level of Major CCs called MCC.

2.13 Resource Level & Skill Planning

- CDI & Coder staffing levels. Identify the levels of coder and CDI staffing and resources required under simulated workload associated with ICD-10. Provide reports of expected workload and resource requirements by specialty and service lines.
- Areas where additional physician documentation will be necessary. Identify under-documentation by specialty, by physician and diagnosis categories.

2.14 ICD-9 to ICD-10 Documentation Improvement/Opportunities

- Identify the financial and reimbursement impact based on documentation improvement to CMI benchmark level. Provide these reports by service line with drill down capability to individual physician, by specialty and by patient demographics.
- Risk Level Identification. Identify and reports on risks associated with under-documentation. Clinical Intelligence tools can provide risk level of requiring additional documentation for ICD-10 by physician (both attending and operating physician roles), by specialty and by patient demographics. Reports can identify risk level of new documentation elements necessary in ICD-10 including laterality, acuity, anatomical location, combination and complication codes. Risk levels associated with unspecified code utilization by specialty and by physician (both attending and operating) can be analyzed using Clinical Intelligence tools.
- Gap Analysis. Clinical Intelligence methods can identify gaps in coding and documentation between ICD-9 and ICD-10. Given the current ICD-9 level of documentation, the gap analysis can identify where documentation and coding are insufficient to meet those required by ICD-10 level. The gap analysis can provide reports of documentation gaps by categories of:
  - Acuity,
  - Anatomic location,
  - Laterality,
  - Combination and complication codes by specialty, medical unit, physician (both attending and operation physician roles)
- Documentation "gap" report can be based on medical claims data analysis by service line, specialty, patient demographics, payer and physician (both attending and operating physician roles).
- Hospital Safety Analytics. Based on coding information and claims data, it's possible to provide analysis and reports on hospital patient safety indicators. By using differential analysis of patient DRG codes and Present on Arrival (POA) codes, the analyst can determine which codes were added as Hospital Acquired Complications (HAC). This information can be grouped via classification algorithms, or can be included in statistical analysis to generate trend lines (regression analysis), categorized by service line, patient demographics and other metrics. Analytics can determine the losses incurred due to HAC and can provide the basis for return on investment in improving patient safety practices to reduce HAC.

2.15 Clinical Intelligence for Utilization Management and Review

Clinical Intelligence can help daily reviews of admissions that include key review diagnosis and accelerate clinical care team decision. Using Clinical Intelligence reports, or dashboards, the Utilization Review Team and/or Case Managers review the daily admissions that include key review diagnoses. It can also ensure the documentation is accurate and that medical necessity is well-documented.

These Clinical Intelligence tools make it possible for Case Managers to be alerted of important factors during treatment, as well as throughout the discharge planning process, without having to read through pages of documentation.

The Clinical Intelligence tools can easily use filters to identify "patients of interest". For example, some of these filters could be set up to identify patients with the following clinical conditions:

- Patients with high CHADS2 & CHA2SD2 VASc Scores[25]
- Patients with high ABCD2 Scores[26]. Locate all patients with an ABCD2 score of 3 or higher, concurrently or retrospectively
- Patients with specific HAS-BLED Scores[27]
- Patients that meet Pneumonia Severity Index Scores

2.16 Clinical Pathways

A patient who presents with certain symptoms is diagnosed during a visit but two other opportunities to treat the patient are missed: first what other checks and procedures can be applied while patient is in the office? For example, should the patient be vaccinated, blood drawn for annual test, or other test that apply to the patient based on the patient's demographics and prior medical history. Second, once patient is diagnosed, what is the proper sequence of treatment protocol and forward-looking schedule of appointments necessary to move the patient through the diverse care providers. For example, when a patient presents with a problem, a sequence of tests, referrals and follow-up appointments may be indicated.

This application provides a graphical path that illustrates for care provider the sequence of care episodes necessary to completely treat patient to recovery and maximize the types of care to patient while patient comes in for each visit.

Building a clinical pathways application uses a set of pre-defined clinical decision tree templates. These templates are created based on a combination of propensity analytics on clinical or claims data (discharge data can also be used) to incorporate best practices from applicable empirical care protocols. (See an example of clinical decision tree in Part II under Case Based Reasoning section). These models could be periodically updated (monthly?) reflecting any new trends in the data. The models could also be particularized based on categories (hospital size, type, location, patient demographics, etc.), as indicated by the data to be statistically significant. Furthermore, each hospital would be able to modify its decision tree if so desired. An HL7 interface (ADT & notes & Lab results, etc.) to the EMR provides input to the application. The real-time application would suggest the schedule and sequence of treatments.

---

[25] CHADS2 calculates patient risk of stroke with AFIB. CHADS2 VASc includes additional vascular parameters in the calculation.
[26] ABCD2 score is a clinical score to determine the risk for stroke within the first two days following a transient ischemic attack (TIA).
[27] HAS-BLED score is a clinical score used for assessing bleeding risk in patients with atrial fibrillation (AF).

2.17 Osteopathic prediction model

Many patients present with ailments from musculoskeletal (MSK) issues, including osteopenia and osteoporosis. In addition, issues related to osteonecrosis are serious conditions that should be known to physicians before performing procedures. Certain patients have MSK markers and pre-conditions related to bone density and localized bone problems that disqualify them for certain procedures. For example a patient who suffers from osteonecrosis is not a good candidate for dental implant or requires extra caution for joint replacement procedures.

Our goals is to develop an application that offers predictive scores of patient musculoskeletal markers indicating whether patient should be further tested for osteopenia or osteonecrosis and whether there are precautions about performing procedures on that patient.

To build this application you need to ingest one year prior patient history and diagnostics lab or radiology results associated with patient MSK tests, other demographics, life style and patient health status (smoker, blood test results, etc.) to train a predictive model. When a patient is registered or admitted, patient's data is ingested via HL7 interface and the application provides an osteo-musculoskeletal precaution score.

2.18 Decision support system for Antibiotic prescription

Patients acquire infection complications during their stay in hospitals. These infections pose the government and hospitals a huge cost that is avoidable. Whether a particular protocol for treating patients with antibiotics is the right approach is often an open question. Furthermore, we have an incomplete understanding of patient populations, patient reaction to certain antibiotics, and the efficacy of those antibiotics in treating the condition without creating adverse effects. In addition, new antibiotic agents are released and recommended for different types of diseases which are documented in the IDSA database, but are not always known to the physician at the point of care.

The application recommends antibiotic prescriptions, based on the patient's history and their current condition, as well as an up-to-date antibiotic database and a model of patient reactions to antibiotics. This can equip the physician with better decision support in making antibiotic prescriptions. In the long run, this can also curb the overall cost of treatment for hospital-acquired infections.

In order to build this application, first Ingest several years (or all of) prior patient medical history (EMRs) including allergy and precaution data. Ingest the IDSA database and build a real-time interface to the IDSA database. Build a model of antibiotic interactions in patients, and update this based on new patient histories and new antibiotics. When patient is admitted to the ER or as inpatient, the application can suggest the appropriate antibiotic based on patients' prior history of reaction or response to prior antibiotic prescription and based on IDSA's recommended antibiotic type.

2.19 Antibiotic tracking & alert system

Often patient infections don't respond properly to an antibiotic because the specific antibiotic agent is ineffective for the particular infection, but also often because the prescribed antibiotic is not administered on time and/or at the correct dose (Right dose, Right Time).

This application tracks patient's stay in hospital from pre-surgery to post-op and recovery, continuously reconciling the physician's antibiotic prescriptions and the time and doze of administration. When discrepancies are detected, such cases are flagged as alerts.

For building this application, you can start with a HL7 interface to the EMR tracks the physician antibiotic prescription and regular nurse/PA charts that indicate when the antibiotic was administered, the route (IV, oral, etc.) and dose. Often discrepancies occur when a patient is not given the antibiotic, or given the antibiotic at the wrong time or wrong dose, or when physician has discontinued the antibiotic but the nurse continues to administer the antibiotic.

2.20 PTSD & Suicide prediction application

Often, patients admitted to the ER for trauma care experience post traumatic disorders. Such disorders go unchecked leading to post-traumatic problems for patients. Additionally, many patients with behavioral health complications or prior suicide (or self-injury) attempts go unnoticed. The goal of this application is to predict the severity of PTSD in patients and predict which patients are at risk of self-harm.

The goal of this application is that it interfaces to the EMR or ER charting system and is able to predict which trauma patients are likely to experience PTSD complications or risk of suicide which require further referral for mental health/behavioral health visits with specialists. This application is not for diagnosis but for providing a measure of risk. The users are physicians in ER, hospitalists or family physicians who have access to patient medical records and can apply the application as a decision support system.

Building this application requires that a prediction engine be trained using prior hospital data and national databases to build predictive models specific to PTSD prediction. The application is able to take EMR notes and coded information (ICD-9, ICD-10 or DSM-IV or DSM-V) to build a data-driven predictive model.

2.21 Clinical prediction rules & decision support system

Prior research and clinical trials produce a set of rubrics and heuristics known as Clinical Prediction Rules. When simplified into decision rules, physician use these rules to make clinical decisions. For example, the Geneva rule is a guideline that computes a score that determines if a patient is at risk for DVT/PE. Similarly, the Ottawa rule determines in case a patient experiences joint injury, if an X-ray exam is justified.

To address this challenge, a rule-based decision tree application can automatically compute clinical prediction rules for patients and flag any alerts for each patient.

How does the application work? The application ingests prior EMR data and uses a library of clinical prediction rules to provide scores for various tests and clinical decision making. The application is able to use unsupervised learning to generate a rule-based engine that can generate rules specific to the patient population.

2.22 Intelligent Eligibility check

When patients present or are admitted to hospital, the common assumption is that their insurance provider is current and they're eligible for insurance coverage or they have adequate insurance coverage. Often the patient eligibility is not checked upfront or when checked, it requires lots of manual effort. Similarly, when a patient arrives to ER, hospital or clinic, the patient is unaware of their financial responsibility for the treatment that they're about to receive.

Envision this application to be connected to the payers can determine if the patient is eligible for the treatment that they're about to receive and determine what is the patient's financial share of the obligation. This eligibility check can happen instantly and quickly. This solution helps hospitals and clinical avoid payment issues and denials with payers. Another feature of the application can obtain electronic pre-authorization from the payer if that payer requires pre-authorization for the treatment/exam or procedure. The benefit is higher payment and reimbursement for the care providers.

Building this application requires an HL7 interface (ADT and Insurance payer segments) to the provider's EMR system allows patient information to flow into the application. The application maintains a link to the insurance providers to check patient's eligibility and also perform pre-authorization when necessary.

2.23 Treatment costing program

One of the CMS triple aims is for care providers to reduce costs. This aim has been handled in large and broad scale by care providers, but most are unable to track costs on a per treatment or per case basis. Without knowing the cost basis for their products (exams, treatments, procedures, etc.), it is nearly impossible to know which specific cost-cutting areas to target. Some hospitals are working to reduce costs by minimizing their supply costs. This is helpful but does not cover the operational costs.

This application would provide an activity-based costing application can compute and analyze cost of procedures, tests and treatments by patient, by physician and several other factors producing costing models and dashboards. Such models can provide the detailed cost variances and pricing necessary to maintain a desired margin.

The application ingests and integrates data from the care provider's charge master, supply chain cost, inventory data, EMR records, CPT/ICD9 codes, patient activity (ADT time stamps) to build the costing model. The model can present distribution curves using descriptive statistics to highlight the norm and outliers. It can use unsupervised pattern recognition engine to identify patterns and root causes in cost overruns. The application can use the engine to identify opportunities for cost reduction.

2.24 Clinical Decision Support System

The gold standard for referrals and tests is often not consistent among practice sites and among physicians. A set of best practices for appropriateness of physician decisions such as referring to specialists, orders for exams and tests (such as lab tests, cardiac tests, GI exams, radiology scans, etc.) are compiled by several organizations including the ACR (American College of Radiology), ABIM (American Board of Internal Medicine), etc.

A decision support application makes recommendations as to the appropriateness of a physician's order for follow-up test or visits. The application uses standard guidelines from ACR, ABIM and other acknowledged sources of guidelines. This application promises to reduce the frequency of over-used or abused procedures and exams, thereby reducing costs and investing medical decision making with greater consistency and appropriateness, ultimately improving patient care.

To build this application, it requires the application to have ADT (Admit, Discharge, Transfer) data and medical history information for a patient by ingesting prior EMR medical notes and patient demographic data. When a doctor enters a diagnosis and then an order (for a test, or referral, or exam, etc.), the application scores the decision based on the criteria captured in the rule-based engine trained by the best practices guidelines. The appropriateness of each decision can be shown by Red (inappropriate), Yellow (additional information is needed in order to determine if the case meets the procedure's criteria) and green (appropriate). If Red or Yellow indicators are presented, the doctor can enter additional justifications if required to re-score his/her decision.

Clinical analytics offers numerous opportunities for improving patient care outcomes, patient health population and reduce cost of care across the entire care continuum. We now have the broadest and most complete collection of analytics engines including concept extraction (Natural language processing supported by medical dictionaries and advanced inferencing), optimization engine, predictive modeling engine, classifiers, pattern recognition engine that finds insights and patterns from data, machine learning, and Inferencing engine that allows rule-based deductive and inductive reasoning.

Some of the additional advanced clinical analytics solutions are explained in the next sections:

2.25 Computerized Auto-Coding (CAC) suite of applications.

These applications automatically translate and map content from medical notes and assign ICD-9, ICD-10, HCPCS, CPT codes plus applying Grouper and Local Edit rules. Other variations of this application provide audits of previously coded notes to determine whether the codes assigned were correct or the medical note was under-coded or over-coded. These applications are based on several analytical components and stages of analytics that use a trained coding engine.

A coding engine is a form of analytical classifier. The data scientist takes one to two years of historical medical notes and associated codes from claims data to train the engine. The coding engine learns from prior data and builds internal hard-wiring between text and codes. The more data is available, the higher accuracy of the coding engine.

In the first state, chart abstraction approach that allows extracting structured concepts from unstructured data (medical notes) is applied. Chart abstracting starts by dividing a medical note into its main sections such as Findings, History, Diagnosis and other sections in the note. Using over 100 medical dictionaries such as UMLS, LOINC, MeSH, MTH, SNOMED and by using Natural Language Processing (NLP) technology, the chart abstraction component is able to extract relevant terms from the note and discern the type of those terms. For example, it can determine the category of text, if the term is a diagnosis, disease, medication, procedure, lab result, an activity, sign and symptom or other category of text.

In the next stage, the inferencing component determines the polarity of the text. Inferencing is a form of artificial intelligence that can reason about something. Here the inferencing component determines whether the extracted terms is positive or negative, whether it's speculative, conditional or hypothetical. This step is critical in defining what terms are positive and the confidence in the truth about the text.

In the 3rd stage, the CAC assigns a code from ICD-9 or ICD-10 to the term and then using inferencing again determines the primary versus secondary diagnosis. During a coding session, as the coding engine suggests codes to a coder for each note, the coder can modify the code by removing or adding a new code. The correcting step provides feedback to the engine and acts as a supervised training to the auto-coding engine. Finally in the last stage, using rule-based methods the coding engine applies Grouper rules, and local edits to complete the coding process.

The application can measure the confidence score for each code that is automatically assigned. Typically, when the confidence level is high, you can decide to send the claim directly to billing without a human coder review. You can set a threshold level of confidence, for example, all medical notes with confidence level of 95% or higher, can be directly sent to billing. This process is called direct-to-bill. The more accurate your CAC application, the higher volume of your medical notes will be in the direct-to-bill category.

The advantages of CAC include higher coder productivity, higher coding accuracy and higher coding consistency across the enterprise.

2.26 Re-admission Prediction.

This application uses predictive modeling in a novel way. There are two approaches to making prediction. One method uses the rule-based approaches such as LACE. LACE stands for Length of Stay, Acuity, Comorbidity and ED visits. Prior research using regression analysis based on certain patient populations have provided clues to the predictors and markers associated to patient re-admission to hospitals. The LACE method offers a simple rubric to compute a re-admission score for any patient after discharge from hospital. Such approaches, while grounded in scientific research, are not adequately accurate and not generalizable. While the results are always interesting, such approaches produce a high volume of False Positives (FP) and False Negatives (FN). The reasons are that research that produced the rules, typically worked with a limited patient population and was limited a geographic location. The third reason is a termporal reason. The research was done a while ago and over time people's health and disease characteristics change. Hence, the rule-based approaches and evidence-based methods are only a good baseline to start from and never the end goal.

The data-driven approaches specifically use predictive models on the data collected from a relevant patient population. These models use unsupervised learning from past data to detect associations and insight from the data. The data can come from a specific patient population for a hospital or geography. Unlike the rule-based approaches that are static, the data driven predictive models are adaptive. They can always update themselves and adapt as new data is incorporated in the predictive model. Hence their accuracy is much higher.

We use the rule-based approach to establish a base line to measure the accuracy in terms of the number of False Positives (FP) and False Negatives (FN), but then we use data-driven approaches, the predictive modeling methods to improve accuracy. For example, a re-admission prediction application showed that using predictive modeling methods that incorporated ensemble models and signal boosting were up to 40% in re-admission prediction that the LACE method.

Predictive medicine can include a number of other use cases. The application is able to determine which inpatients are likely to experience hospital acquired complications such as DVT/PE or Sepsis and infections, adverse events and falls. In behavioral health area, the application can provide suicide predictions and models that can foretell which patients are at risk of self-harm. Using these sophisticated predictive modeling approaches, we can predict which children are likely to have autism or other syndromes.

Re-admission prediction provides which patients are likely to be readmitted after discharge. This approach offers the opportunity to prevent readmissions. On average 30% of readmissions can be prevented. On average, using re-admission prediction can save a hospital as much as $5M in avoidable medical expenses, let alone that the patients are spared from unnecessary medical treatment at readmissions.

2.27 Behavioral Health Analytics.

Behavioral health is one of the most promising applications of clinical analytics. Using analytics, we're able to determine correlations between behavioral health diagnosis, medications and outcomes. For example, we can track health of patients who are on two or more anti-psychotic drugs. We can correlate patient's medical and behavioral data together and use non-linear logistic regression to identify predictors of outcomes. We're able to use the same data to train classification engines (classifiers) to classify patients into various disease categories or suggest various care protocols. The diagnostic codes used in behavioral health are DSM IV and DSM V standards, but there are direct cross-walks between these codes and ICD-9/ICD-10 codes. There are opportunities to predict self-injury and suicide (as mentioned above) and determine the markers that indicate a patient's mental health progression through the course of care.

2.28 Health Cost Utilization.

This application provides a view into a hospital's internal costs and revenues. It ingests claims data as a starting point, but can also include ADT (Admit Discharge Transfer) data to analyze the activities that generate revenue for the hospital and contrast those with activities that are responsible for costs. The analysis gives hospital administrators insight into the resource utilization in their organization. The claims data when analyzed are excellent source of information about care providers (physicians), departments, procedures and patient population. The dasbhoards show how hospital sources of revenues by specialty, physicians or physician groups, by patient population, by disease and by other demographic factors. The cost analysis can be extracted from the purchasing and financial system. The financial system provides clues to the cost of labor, FTEs (Full Time Equivalent) personnel resources consumed and supplies purchased by department and more granular activity. The more granular the data the better accuracy in allocating cost to activities and better insight in comparison costs to revenues. Using this application, hospitals can discern what programs are profitable and which activities represent losses.

Using ADT data, we're able to show where hospital operations are experiencing waste. One of the inherent and telling patterns in ADT data is the frequently that patients are transferred between various departments or hospital locations. The frequency and the degree that patients are transferred back-and-forth can be telltales of inefficiency in hospital operations. Similarly, once there is access to the hospital's patient scheduling data, we can analyze and present dashboards about operational efficiency of that hospital. The frequency that patient visits and procedures get rescheduled, regardless of inpatient or outpatient status, can provide measures of operational efficiency. In addition, using this data, we can provide utilization measures to show how efficiently hospital resources and healthcare capacity are being utilized. These measures can point out waste and inefficiency in areas and practices that the hospital can address.

2.29 Physician referral patterns.

This application shows the physician referral patterns for a hospital starting the physicians outside of the hospital affiliations and how those referrals connect to the hospital's specialists and eventually to the procedures performed. This graphical representation illustrates the network diagram of who refers patients to whom and the chain of referral. The importance of this application is for hospitals to understand the referral patterns that are sources of patient and revenues to their hospital. Armed with this information, hospitals can focus their marketing and public relations programs at targeted physicians groups and patient population more effectively.

2.30 Population Health Management.

This suite of applications come with interactive analytics dashboards that allow public health professionals, care providers (physicians and nursing staff) and other clinical staff to track patient population by their disease and provide health coaching to improve their health. Population health management analytics classifies patient population by age, gender, zip code (or county boundaries) and other demographics, by disease and comorbidities, by progression of the disease, by sign and symptoms and other clinical measures such as vaccination data.

These applications display geographic map dashboards that show the concentration and movement of population with certain chronic condition. Some of the use-cases for example include a hospitalist use who wants to identify their diabetic and pre-diabetic patient population. The query produces the results in a graphical dashboard. The user can drill down on the map to find specific patients in the population. In other use cases, a user might search for all patients over 60 who have missed their immunization or identify patient population with prior cardiac heart failure.

Similarly, a hospitalist might be interested to know the progression of pre-diabetic patients by age groups (pre-teen, teen, adult, etc.), tracking the population's BMI (Bio-Mass Index) and other markers to determine how the population health is changing. Tracking community health progression is key to estimate trends and predictions about the future health costs of a population.

2.31 Patient engagement applications.

These applications strive to engage patients in their health by promoting better diet, exercise and balanced work-life behaviors. These applications consist of two components: a patient-facing application and an analytics engine in the back-end. Through the patient-facing interface, these applications typically invite the user to a web portal or a smart phone app where the patient records their food intake, activity level and their signs and symptoms. Often the patient-facing portal allows integration of data from other wearable devices such as a Fitbit.

The analytics engine in the back-end is able to classify patients based on the aggregation of this data and provide a number of results, alerts and messages. The analytics engine correlates the patient's data with their disease conditions across the entire population and identify abnormal and outlier patients. The engine can use a rule-based approach to send alerts and messages to the patient if patient's data meets certain rule or exceeds certain threshold (such as BMI level). It can notify the primary care physician or the patient's health coach of such alerts. In addition, the analytics engine can identify which tactics, messaging and programs are effective on which category of patient population. The overall benefit of using patient engagement application is prevention and reduction of preventable ER visits. This application promises to reduce cost of care and improve patient population health. When combined with the patient population health management system, it can provide a wealth of information about patient health demographics and cost of care. Insurance companies are eager to use these applications in order to curb their costs.

2.32 Fraud-Waste-Abuse Applications

The Federal government has enabled CMS to combat fraud and fraudulent reimbursement claims. The CMS is required to fight fraud with technologies such as predictive modeling. Using predictive analytics, CMS is able to collect data for relevant factors and predictors to predict the likelihood of a claim being accurate. The models use logistic regression and neural networks to make predictions and classifications.

CMS has contracted with RAC audit companies to detect and recover from fraudulent medical claims, but the outcome has produced mixed results. While the volume of detected suspicious claims has been higher than expected, the success rate of recovery has lagged due to lack of high precision analytics. Several companies have been successful in Fraud-Waste-Abuse detection due to the ability to apply both rule-based and unsupervised data mining. An analytics application can detect suspicious claims based on CMS guidelines for correct coding. These guidelines include rules that require appropriateness checks: does the procedure (CPT) code match the diagnosis (ICD-9/ICD-10) code? Does the procedure (CPT) code match the patient gender, age and demographic? Is this claim a duplicate or is the procedure not plausible? (for example, a medical claim for an appendectomy procedure for a patient that has had a prior appendectomy).

The supervised methods use the CMS rules to identify which claims are suspicious. The unsupervised approach allows for the data to "speak" for itself. The unsupervised data uses clustering and classification models to identify how physician's claims compare to their peers.

The analysis takes several stages: First, the data scientist defines a persona around providers by the type of ICD diagnosis and procedures in their claims. The data scientist defines the personas using classification models. These personas can identify groups of physicians. For example, neurosurgeons would group together while orthopedic surgeons would cluster around their own group. The groups are automatically identified using classifiers. In the second stage, once the members of the group are labeled, the data scientist is able to compare each provider's claims to his/her peers. The engine can identify the frequency of claims, the norm, median and standard deviation of each group's claims. The engine then compares each provider's claims with other members' claims in the group. By performing these comparisons for each provider, we can identify outliers and abnormal claims that fall outside of 3-sigma or higher. This is the basis of unsupervised anomaly and outlier detection in fraud-waste and abuse applications.

2.33 ACO measures - Quality Measures.

A number of healthcare quality organizations are working to define healthcare outcome quality measures and metrics. These organizations include the Leapfrog Group, NQF (National Quality Forum), National Association of Healthcare Quality (NAHQ), the American Health Quality Association(AHQA), Agency for Health Research and Quality (AHRQ) and other organizations such as World Alliance for Patient Safety, the Joint Commission on

Accreditation of Healthcare Organizations (JCAHO) and the Health Foundation in the UK publish quality metrics that together can come to 1,000 measurements. The Accountable Care Organization (ACO) model proposed by CMS uses 33 quality measures (as of 2014), but the number of measures are likely to increase to 64 and higher in the coming years.

These measures typically consist of ratios computed from numerator and denominator values. Typically, the denominator represents total number of patients that meet certain criteria (such as a disease or procedure). The numerator represents the total number of patients that did not receive the proper, standard of care. For example, ACO measure #14 is a ratio of patients who have received their influenza immunization divided by the total patient population cared for by the institution. Similarly, ACO measure #21 is a quality measure about patients with high blood pressure. It's numerator is the number of patients classified as having high blood pressure who were screened by a provider and the provider documented a follow-up. The denominator is the total number of patients with high blood pressure who were being cared for by the provider.

The CMS guidelines have elaborate inclusions and exclusions which require careful translation of the rules into analytics models in order to compute the ratios correctly. Many of these quality measures can be computed automatically once the data becomes available. The minimum dataset required includes patient demographics including master patient index, visit number and claims data that can be mapped to each patient visit.

2.34 Revenue Leakage Analytics

There is an opportunity to build analytics models for medical revenue intelligence, detecting and correcting revenue leakage for medical coding and billing applications. Using the leakage analysis solution, you can improve efficiency, reimbursements and provides analytical insight into organizational revenue capture performance on core measures such as medical coding accuracy, coder productivity, physician documentation problems, clinical outcomes, ,and coding errors and anomalies. Using analytics models a computer program can detect under-coding, over-coding, and mis-coding. An analytics application can also ensure that documentation is consistent with codes.

The Center for Medicaid Services (CMS) has reported losses over $64billion to improper payments. In its investigation of 79 acute care hospitals, the OIG has recovered almost $34 million. The improper and inaccurate billing costs both the CMS in improper payments and costs the hospitals in fines and audit expenses. The revenue leakage analyzer can prevent and identify these problems using specialized analytics.

The revenue Leakage Analyzer provides an automatic and central view to discordance in medical coded claims. It works by automatically extracting concepts (such as diagnoses, procedures, symptoms, allergies, treatments, drugs, body parts, laterality, etc.) from the text in clinical encounter notes such as physician notes, lab results, and admit/discharge records, and uses these concepts to infer codes — including ICD-10. The solution provides a report of possible discrepancies between codes sent to the billing system and the correctly justifiable codes. xPatterns Revenue Leakage Analyzer flags non-compliance in records – such as violations in CCI edits, MUE edits. It also checks for inconsistencies between diagnosis and procedure codes and confirms that codes entered in a billing system have justifying documentation in an encounter. Additionally, it reports how a doctor's E/M levels compare to the national CMS-reported averages.

2.35 Revenue Prediction Analytics

Predicting revenue and cash position is of interest to financial managers in hospitals. Most medical Claims are paid right away and the rest go through a pending status where they might be denied, then re-submitted and eventually appealed by the provider to receive payment. There is a need for providers to know how much and when they'll receive payment. Similarly, what is the patient responsibility given the patient's payer and eligibility level for a given treatment/procedure.

This analytics application has the analytics capability that provides revenue projection dashboards showing the expected and risk-adjusted value of receivables and claims filed by the provider. The dashboards show projected revenue by patient classification, payer and procedures. The application uses payment history to analyze projected and risk-adjusted payments over a future (for example 30-120 days) time horizon. The application can analyze payment history retrospectively to show outliers related to certain procedures, payers and types of claims. At the patient level, the application can show patient's financial responsibility before a procedure is performed. The application would also show comparison of payer's payments on procedures and in general for each provider so the provider can compare the provider's claim payment performance against his/her peers on a specific procedure or across an entire practice.

Chapter 3: Clinical Data Sets: Content & Registries

The following datasets and clinical registries are likely desirable content to be integrated into your clinical intelligence analytics or clinical research. These databases are alphabetically listed[28]. There are additional databases that available through grant funding and other research institutions. A good source of access to many of these databases is www.bridgetodata.org, and HIMSS publications.

Clinical Dataset / Registry	Description - Source
ADIS	Covers pharmaceutical evidence-based research and drug safety database. It includes drugs in pipeline for final trial and can evaluate products in development or upcoming drugs. It's offered by Wolters Kluwer Pharma Solutions.
AERS	FDA - Adverse Event Reporting System (AERS)
BIOSIS	Biological abstracts, part of Life Sciences in the Web of Knowledge, covers life sciences abstracts and citation indexing. Owned by Thomas Reuters.
BRFSS	Behavioral Risk Factor Surveillance System
CPRD	Clinical Practice Research Datalink is the new National Institute of Health (NIH)
CARDIA	Coronary Artery Risk Development in Young Adults Study
CDB/RM	University HealthSystem Consortium (UHC) Clinical Database/Resource Manager (CDB/RM)
CHS	Cardiovascular Health Study
CEA	Cost-Effectiveness Analysis (CEA) Registry
Cerner Health Facts	Cerner Health Facts Database
CINAHL	Cumulative Index to Nursing and Allied Health Services
DAWN	Drug Abuse Warning Network (DAWN)
EMBASE	A database of 25million literature records for pharma/drug vigilance to comply with regulations, deep drug indexing, tracking drug adverse events in literature. Produced by Elsevier.
ENCODE	Encyclopedia of DNA Elements, an international consortium database to collect data on human genome project, human gene proteins and RNAs.
Entrez	National Center for Biotechnology Information (NCBI) database of human genome project plus other databases for genetic genotypes and phenotype correlations called dbGaP.
HPRD	Human Protein Reference Database, a visual database of human proteins.
ICTRP	International Clinical Trials Registry Platform (ICTRP) offered by the World Health Organization maintains a registry of worldwide clinical trials.
IMS Health	Database of therapy and drug effectiveness. IMS LifeLink™ Health Plan Claims Database (formerly PharMetrics Patient-Centric Database)
IntrinsiQ	IntrinsiQ Database
LTC	Analyticare Long Term Care database

---

[28] All trademarks belong to their respective owners.

LRx	IMS LifeLink™ Longitudinal Rx (LRx) Database
MarketScan	MarketScan Commercial Claims and Encounters and offers MarketScan for Medicaid Database
MEPS	Medical Expenditure Panel Survey (MEPS)
MEDS	Medi-Cal Paid Claims Files and statistics published by CMS and state governments.
MediGuard	MediGuard (formerly iGuard)
MeSH	Medical Subject Headings (MeSH), a vocabulary of indexing life sciences journal articles used by PubMed and NLM. The MeSH categories would be a fine list of facets for xPatterns (such as anatomy, diseases, biology, chemicals & drugs, psychiatry, etc).
MIMIC and MIMIC II	One of the largest databases of clinical data about Intensive Care Ujit (ICU) patients. Offered by PhysioNet as free service funded by NIH.
MRFIT	Multiple Risk Factor Intervention Trial (MRFIT)
NBDPN	National Birth Defects Prevention Network (NBDPN)
NAMCS	National Center for Health Statistics: National Ambulatory Medical Care Survey (NAMCS)
NDI	National Death Index (NDI)
NDTI	National Disease and Therapeutic Index (NDTI)
NEISS	National Electronic Injury Surveillance System (NEISS)
NESARC	National Epidemiologic Survey on Alcohol and Related Conditions (NESARC)
NGC Guidelines	Offered by National Guideline Clearinghouse, contains a database of evidence-based medical guidelines.
NHEFS	NHANES I Epidemiologic Followup Study (NHEFS)
NHHCS	National Health Interview Survey (NHIS)
NHHCS	National Home and Hospice Care Survey (NHHCS)
NHAMCS	National Hospital Ambulatory Medical Care Survey (NHAMCS)
NHDS	National Hospital Discharge Survey (NHDS)
NNHS	National Nursing Home Survey (NNHS)
NPDS/TESS	National Poison Data System (NPDS, formerly TESS)
NRDIOSE	National Registry of Drug-Induced Ocular Side Effects (NRDIOSE)
NSCID	National Spinal Cord Injury Database
NSDUH	National Survey on Drug Use and Health (NSDUH)
NSRCF	National Survey of Residential Care Facilities (NSRCF)
NVSS – Birth	National Vital Statistics System (NVSS) contains 3 databases: - Birth Data (CDC), Fetal Death Data (CDC), Mortality Data (CDC)
NARCOMS	North American Research Committee on Multiple Sclerosis (NARCOMS) Registry
OMIM	Online Mendelian Inheritance in Man is a tool used by geneticists. Includes locations of genes, disorders and traits. Must support the OMIM numbering system. Equivalent of the Human Genome Project.
PACE	Pharmaceutical Assistance Contract for the Elderly (PACE)
PCORI	Patient Centered Outcomes Research Institute DB, a new database by Agency for Healthcare Research & Quality (AHRQ)

	to disseminate clinical research results for better clinical decisions.
PPCD	Pharmetrics Patient-Centric Database
Premier-i3	Premier-i3 Continuum of Care Database. Offered by Optum Insight.
PSN	University HealthSystem Consortium (UHC) Patient Safety Net (PSN®)
Pubmed	By National Library of Medicine, includes MEDLINE and NLM database of indexed citation & abstracts. Need ability to link out to free full text articles in other databases. Always show the article's PMID number.
RMRS	Regenstrief Medical Record System (RMRS) database – University of Indiana
REP	Rochester Epidemiology Project (REP) (Mayo Clinic)
SAGE	Systematic Assessment of Geriatric drug use via Epidemiology (SAGE) Database
SCOPUS	One of the largest databases of research and academic journals offered by Elsevier with its own search engine.
SEER	Surveilance, Epidemiology, End Results database. Includes cancer registries that allows statistical analysis on its data.
STDSS	Sexually Transmitted Diseases Surveillance System (STDSS)
Slone Epidemiology Unit	Slone Epidemiology Unit Birth Defects Case Control Study and Surveillance Study
UCSC Genome Browser	A browser that provides visual display of genomics and phenotypes across multiple databases including OMIM, ENCODE and Neandertal.
USRDS	United States Renal Data System (USRDS)
VAERS	FDA - Vaccine Adverse Event Reporting System (VAERS)
VSD	Vaccine Safety Datalink (VSD)

3.1 National Quality Measures

Several organizations such as NQHF and HHS have suggested several quality measures. The list and quantity of measures suggested by these sources are listed below:

- Agency for Healthcare Research & Quality (AHRQ)(182)
- Center for Financing, Access, and Cost Trends (CFACT)(60)
- Administration on Aging (AoA)(9)
- Centers for Disease Control and Prevention (CDC)(136)
- Centers for Medicare & Medicaid Services (CMS)(782)
- Health Resources and Services Administration (HRSA)(148)
- Indian Health Service (IHS)(220)
- National Institutes of Health (NIH)(31)
- Office of the Assistant Secretary for Health (OASH)(491)
- Substance Abuse and Mental Health Services Administration (SAMHSA)(21)

NQF (National Quality Forum) measurement category

National Quality Forum (NQF) measures are divided into two broad categories: Healthcare delivery measures and Population health measures. Each measure is subdivided into specific subcategories of Quality Measures, Related Measures and Efficiency Measures. Figure 3.1 below illustrates the metrics for each subcategory.

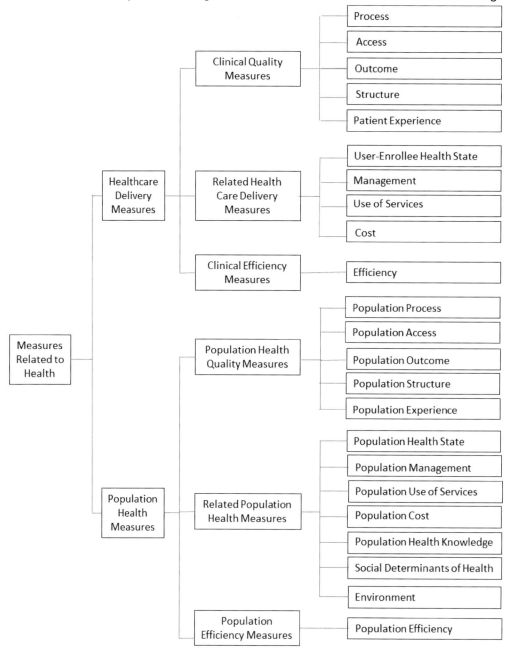

Fig. 3.1 – NQF Quality Measures

The list of these measures can be downloaded from the National Quality Measure Clearing-house (NQMC) at http://www.qualitymeasures.ahrq.gov/hhs-measure-inventory/browse.aspx.

3.2 NQF & CMS Core Measures

The CMS has defined and endorsed over 35 core measures and recommends hospitals to report on these measures routinely. Some of these measures correspond to the measures outlined by National Quality Forum (NQF). The initial core set of quality measures are determined based on recommendations from the Agency for Healthcare Research and Quality's Subcommittee to the National Advisory council for Healthcare Research and Quality and based on public comments. These core set measures will support HHS and its state partners in developing a quality-driven, evidence-based, national system for measuring the quality of healthcare provided to Medicaid-eligible adults. Among these measures a few stand out:

- Flu shots for adults ages 50-64
- Adult BMI [body mass index] assessment
- Plan all-cause readmission
- Diabetes, short-term complications admission rate
- Chronic obstructive pulmonary disease (COPD) admission rate
- Congestive heart failure admission rate
- Follow-up after hospitalization for mental illness
- Comprehensive diabetes care: hemoglobin A1c testing
- Antidepressant medication management
- Adherence to antipsychotic for individuals with schizophrenia
- Care transition—transition record transmitted to health care professional

The more detailed list[29] is shown in Table 3.1 below.

	NQF*	Measure Steward **	Measure Name	Programs in Which the Measure is Currently Used***
Prevention & Health Promotion	0039	NCQA	Flu Shots for Adults Ages 50-64 (Collected as part of HEDIS CAHPS Supplemental Survey)	HEDIS®, NCQA Accreditation,
	N/A	NCQA	Adult BMI Assessment	HEDIS®, Health Homes Core
	0031	NCQA	Breast Cancer Screening	MU1, HEDIS®, NCQA Accreditation, , PQRS GPRO, Shared Savings Program
	0032	NCQA	Cervical Cancer Screening	MU1, HEDIS®, NCQA Accreditation
	0027	NCQA	Medical Assistance With Smoking and Tobacco Use Cessation (Collected as	MU1, HEDIS®, Medicare, NCQA Accreditation

---

[29] Department of Health and Human Services (HHS), Medicaid Program: Initial Core Set of Health Care Quality Measures for Medicaid-Eligible Adults, 01/04/2012. https://s3.amazonaws.com/public-inspection.federalregister.gov/2011-33756.pdf

			part of HEDIS CAHPS Supplemental Survey)	
	0418	CMS	Screening for Clinical Depression and Follow-Up Plan	PQRS, CMS QIP, Health Homes Core, Shared Savings Program
	N/A	NCQA	Plan All-Cause Readmission	HEDIS®
	0272	AHRQ	PQI 01: Diabetes, Short-term Complications Admission Rate	
	0275	AHRQ	PQI 05: Chronic Obstructive Pulmonary Disease (COPD) Admission Rate	Shared Savings Program
	0277	AHRQ	PQI 08: Congestive Heart Failure Admission Rate	Shared Savings Program
	0283	AHRQ	PQI 15: Adult Asthma Admission Rate	
	0033	NCQA	Chlamydia Screening in Women age 21-24 *(same as CHIPRA core measure, however, the State would report on the adult age group)*	MU1, HEDIS®, NCQA Accreditation, CHIPRA Core
Management of Acute Conditions	0576	NCQA	Follow-Up After Hospitalization for Mental Illness	HEDIS®, NCQA Accreditation, CHIPRA Core, Health Home Core
	0469	HCA, TJC	PC-01: Elective Delivery	HIP QDRP, TJC's ORYX Performance Measurement Program
	0476	Prov/C WISH/N PIC/QA S/TJC	PC-03 Antenatal Steroids	TJC's ORYX Performance Measurement Program
Management of Chronic Conditions	0403	NCQA	Annual HIV/AIDS medical visit	
	0018	NCQA	Controlling High Blood Pressure	MU1, HEDIS®, NCQA Accreditation, PQRS GPRO, Shared Savings Program
	0063	NCQA	Comprehensive Diabetes Care: LDL-C Screening	MU1, HEDIS®, NCQA Accreditation, PQRS
	0057	NCQA	Comprehensive Diabetes Care: Hemoglobin A1c Testing	MU1, HEDIS®, NCQA Accreditation, PQRS
	0105	NCQA	Antidepressant Medication Management	MU1, HEDIS®, NCQA Accreditation

	N/A	CMSQMHAG	Adherence to Antipsychotics for Individuals with Schizophrenia	VHA
	0021	NCQA	Annual Monitoring for Patients on Persistent Medications	HEDIS®, NCQA Accreditation
Family Experiences of Care	0006 & 0007	AHRQ & NCQA	CAHPS Health Plan Survey v 4.0 - Adult Questionnaire *with* CAHPS Health Plan Survey v 4.0H - NCQA Supplemental	HEDIS®, NCQA Accreditation, Shared Savings Program (NQF#0006)
Care Coordination	648	AMA-PCPI	Care Transition – Transition Record Transmitted to Health care Professional	Health Homes Core
Availability	0004	NCQA	Initiation and Engagement of Alcohol and Other Drug Dependence Treatment	MU1, HEDIS®, Health Homes Core
	1391	NCQA	Prenatal and Postpartum Care: Postpartum Care Rate *(second component to CHIPRA core measure "Timeliness of Prenatal Care," State would now report 2/2 components instead of 1)*	HEDIS®

Table 3.1 – List of Key Quality Measures

*NQF ID:

- National Quality Forum identification numbers are used for measures that are NQF-endorsed; otherwise, NA is used.

**Measure Steward:

- AHRQ – Agency for Healthcare Research and Quality
- CMS – Centers for Medicare & Medicaid Services
- CMS-QMHAG – Centers for Medicare & Medicaid Services, Quality Measurement and Health Assessment Group
- HCA, TJC – Hospital Corporation of America-Women's and Children's Clinical Services, The Joint
- Commission
- NCQA –National Committee for Quality Assurance
- Prov/CWISH/NPIC/QAS/TJC – Providence St. Vincent Medical Center/Council of Women's and
- Infant's Specialty Hospitals/National Perinatal Information Center/Quality Analytic Services/The Joint
- Commission
- TJC – The Joint Commission

***Programs in which Measures currently are in Use:

- CHIPRA Core – Children's Health Insurance Program Reauthorization Act - Initial Core Set
- CMS QIP – CMS Quality Incentive Program
- HIP QDRP – Hospital Inpatient Quality Data Reporting Program
- Health Homes Core-- CMS Health Homes Core Measures
- MU1 – Meaningful Use Stage 1of the Medicare & Medicaid Electronic Health Record Incentive
- Programs
- PQRS – Physician Quality Reporting Program Group Practice Reporting Option
- Shared Savings Program – Medicare Shared Savings Program
- VHA – Veterans Health Administration

3.3 LeapFrog Measures

Leapfrog is an organization that attempts to measure and improve patient safety and outcomes. The organization gathers and compares measurements from hospitals across four categories: Computer Physician Order Entry (CPOE), ICU Physician Staffing (IPS), Evidence-Based Hospital Referral (EBHR), and eight of the remaining NQF safe practices. Clinical intelligence tools can investigate the root causes of outcomes by determining the underlying factors that are associated with a certain outcome. A list of these measurements is listed below.

CPOE:

1. At least 75% of inpatient medication orders are placed via a computer system that includes decision support software to reduce prescription errors
2. Demonstrate that at least 50% of all common serious prescribing errors in its inpatient CPOE system can be detected and alert physicians on medication checking categories such as drug:drug and drug:allergy interactions.

Evidence-Based Hospital Referral (EBHR) Leap:

There are seven sets of measurements that the Leapfrog organization collects. These measurements focus on high-risk surgical procedures.

1) Coronary artery bypass graft
2) Percutaneous coronary intervention
3) Aortic valve replacement
4) Abdominal aortic aneurysm repair
5) Pancreatic resection
6) Esophagectomy
7) Bariatric Surgery

Common Acute Conditions (CAC):

The measures under this category (or called leaps by the leapfrog organization) address the Acute Myocardial Infarctions (AMI), Pneumonia, and Normal Deliveries.

- Places at or above 80% of the possible quartile scoring points for the NQF-endorsed process-of-care quality measures for the condition as determined by national data

- Places in the two lowest (best) quartiles for resource utilization for the condition treated, as measured by the Adjusted Length of Stay (ALOS).

- Exceeds the specified goal for performance on the nationally-endorsed "Elective Deliveries Before 39 Weeks Gestation" outcome measure and either the "Incidence of Episiotomy" outcome measure or both of the process measures.

3.3 Taxonomy of Clinical Intelligence Dashboards

This chapter provides some use case specifications and details about a typical Clinical Intelligence report and Dashboard utility. The use cases are conceptual, but are detailed enough to give some guidance on what metrics can be tracked, analyzed and reported in dashboards. I'll start by describing the four tiers associated with data reporting in Clinical Intelligence domain. This is a taxonomy of dashboards for healthcare. There are four tiers of drill-down in a typical drill-down scenario:

- *Executive (Enterprise) level* – this is the executive dashboard aggregation of data, a summary across the enterprise and a specific time period. This level also includes dashboards by themes. Goals: strategic
- *Departmental level* – this is the 2nd drill-down tier, to a specific time-line or a dept. level or a particular medical practice. Goal: Decision Support
- *Manager level* – this is the detailed level by an Actor, or an individual type of procedure, or CPT code. Goal: Operational
- *Individual level* – this is the most detailed level of detail, drill-down to the collection of individual EMR records for a patient, or physician, coder. Goal: Audit

The natural progression of user interaction with the report system along these four drill-down levels is depicted in the following graph only as an illustration to show the multiple levels of drill-down and to show that in each level, data may be shown by different styles and types of graphs:

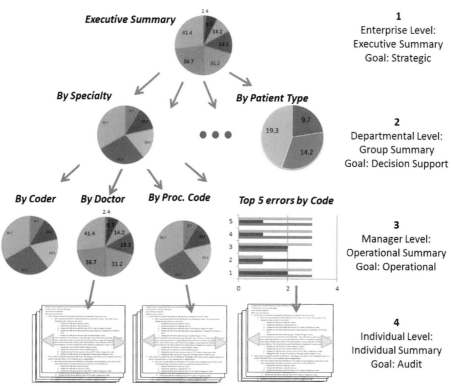

Fig. 3.2 – The Four Level Hierarchy of Analytics Reports

Level descriptions to the right of the figure:

1 — Enterprise Level: Executive Summary / Goal: Strategic

2 — Departmental Level: Group Summary / Goal: Decision Support

3 — Manager Level: Operational Summary / Goal: Operational

4 — Individual Level: Individual Summary / Goal: Audit

3.4 Executive Summary Reports

An Executive summary report shows the high level summary of all data analysis from the Clinical Intelligence program. This is a senior management level report.

The diagram below illustrates the possible fields in an executive Summary Report of a medical coding audit tool:

Summary Findings	Volumes	Financial Impact ($000)	Trend vs. Target
Total no. of Records:	1,000,000	$780,000	⬆
Total No. of Errors Found:	20,000	$140,000	⬆
No. of records under-coded:	15,000	$98,000	⬆
No. of Records with Compliance issues:	2,000	$22,000	⬆
No. of records over-coded:	1,000	$10,000	⬆
No. of records mis-coded:	2,000	$15,000	⬆
Potential Credits	3,000	$2,500	⬇
Potential Revenue Capture	16,000	$110,000	⬆
Potential Net gain (loss)		$107,500	⬆

Table 3.2 – An example of Executive Summary Report for Clinical Coding Audit

Another way to display data is by theme. A theme would define the purpose of the analytics report. Some categories of themes for executive summary reports and dashboards as illustrated next.

Theme #1: Revenue Cycle Theme

The reports for this theme include Hospital Revenue Cycle and Finance Dept. The primary users are Executive, CFO, HIM Manager, End-user Manager. The goal of this report is Strategic.

The report would present the following analytical results:

1. Display the Executive Summary of Clinical Intelligence findings on claims and billing data.
2. Display the results by themes:
    a. Display the top 10 most common under-coded records by CPT code
    b. Display the top 10 most high-dollar records by CPT code
    c. Display the most frequent CPT codes in our records
    d. Display the 20% of codes that represent 80% of the revenues
    e. Display the 20% of codes that represent 80% of under-coding

A graphical Representation of the Executive Summary and the theme summaries can be shows using following Pie charts and Bar charts (Figure 3.3A and 3.3B):

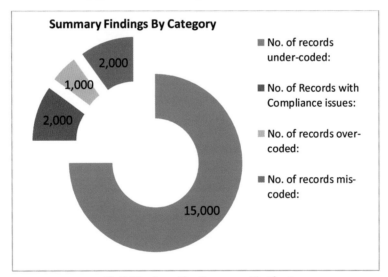

Fig 3.3A - Executive Summary Pie Chart

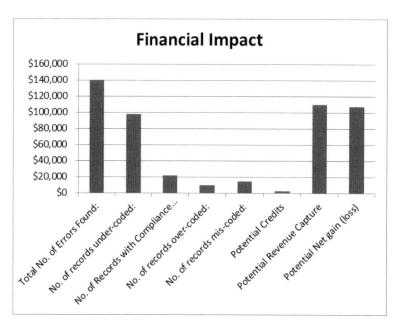

Fig 3.3B - Executive Summary Bar Graph

Theme #2: Cash Flow Projections

The purpose of this repot is to drill down to project cash flow position over the next several months, and the ability to drill down by month or to departmental level (or specialties), as follows:

1. User is able to get cash flow (or projected revenue) summary report. Then clicks on the segments of the pie chart to drill down.
2. User has several options in the drill down to a collection of cases:
   a. To view the drill-down to a portfolio using Time lines. This is shown as a time-series or by a line graph.
   b. To view the drill-down using Sources. This is shown by a pie chart.
      i. Sources can be Medical Specialty, Hospital Unit
   c. A drill down combining the time and source together to show a comparison as month to month by a medical specialty, or hospital unit. This will be shown in a bar graph.

The illustration below shows the possible graph options. The line graph of month-to-month appears in Figure 3.4A. The data by medical specialty (Figure 3.4B) is shown as a pie-of-pie chart.

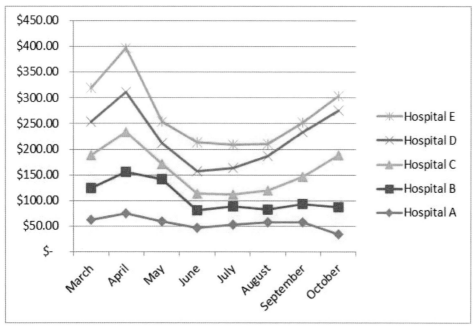

3.4A –Icon of Line Graph for 5 Hospital revenues in a Month to Month Comparison

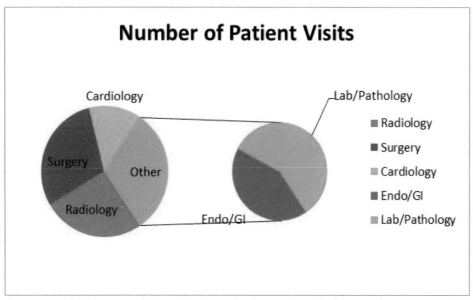

3.4B – Example illustration of Pie-of-pie Chart showing patient visits by specialty

Theme #3: Departmental Performance

The purpose of this report is to drill down to the departmental level, as follows. While the data includes hospital Revenue Cycle and Financial data elements, the theme is around departmental performance. The typical user is a departmental Manager and the goal of this theme is to provide Decision Support. The use-case scenario could follow these steps

1. User clicks on a specific line graph to drill down to a specific time in the chart:
   a. Actor has several options in the drill down to a collection of cases. The results can be displayed as pie charts or a bar chart:
      i. Display the drill-down data by Coders
      ii. Display the drill-down data by Doctors
      iii. Display the drill-down data by class of CPT codes or Diagnosis codes
      iv. Display the drill-down data by patient types (inpatient, Outpatient, ED Patient – EIO)
      v. Display the drill-down data by type of patient length of stay.
   b. User may elect to use themes to view this data. Here, the User is selecting a specific time (say, a particular month or a year) when the Actor clicks on a specific line graph. Then the Actor selects themes by a click on the Theme button, a drop-down list of themes appears (shown below). The Actor selects one of the themes to display the results such as:
      i. Display the top 10 most common data by coders
      ii. Display the top 10 most common data by doctors
      iii. Display the top 10 most common class of CPT codes or diagnostic codes
      iv. Display the data by top 10 categories of longest patient length of stay
2. User clicks on a specific pie slice to drill down. By doing so, the User is narrowing the report to a specific Specialty clinic, or to a medical unit or a department.
   a. Actor has several options for drill down. The results can be displayed as pie charts or bar charts depending on the Actor preference and choice of the Collection:
      i. Display the drill-down data by Coders
      ii. Display the drill-down data by Doctors
      iii. Display the drill-down data by class of CPT codes or Diagnosis codes
      iv. Display the drill-down data by patient types (inpatient, Outpatient, ED Patient – EIO)
      v. Display the drill-down data by type of patient length of stay.
   b. User may elect to use themes to view this data. The User is selecting a specific specialty (for example: Cardiology, Vascular, or Oncology, etc.):
      i. Display the top 10 most common data by coders
      ii. Display the top 10 most common data by doctors
      iii. Display the top 10 most common class of CPT codes or diagnostic codes
      iv. Display the data by top 10 categories of longest patient length of stay
3. Actor clicks on a specific bar chart to drill down to a collection of data in a specific month (or year) and by the specific Clinical Specialty or medical unit. The dashboard displays data according to the User preferences. The Actor selects any one of the following options to display the drill-down collection of data:
      i. Display the drill-down data by Coders
      ii. Display the drill-down data by Doctors
      iii. Display the drill-down data by class of CPT codes or Diagnosis codes
      iv. Display the drill-down data by patient types (inpatient, Outpatient, ED Patient – EIO)
      v. Display the drill-down data by type of patient length of stay.
   b. User may elect to use themes to view this data. The User is selecting a specific specialty (for example: Cardiology, Vascular, or Oncology, etc.):
      i. Display the top 10 most common data by coders

ii. Display the top 10 most common data by doctors

iii. Display the top 10 most common class of CPT codes or diagnostic codes

iv. Display the data by top 10 categories of longest patient length of stay

Theme #4: Individual Performance

The purpose of this theme is to show a use-case for drill downs of analytics to the individual level. The individual level is a collection of data records specific to a physician, a patient, a coder and to other stakeholders in an episode of care. The data includes hospital Revenue Cycle and Financial data. The users include HIM Managers or QI (Quality Improvement) Personnel. The goal of this theme is to perform an audit. The use-case scenario can follow these steps:

1. User clicks on a specific line graph, bar, or slice of pie to drill down further. User can select a number of data categories listed below. Often multiple documents are found which will be shown stacked with the most recent in front. User will page forward or backward in a manner similar behavior to Google ebooks or Kindle. (You can choose and standardize on a single method of paging through multiple EMR records). Actor can drill down to:

    a. Select the related EMR record or records. The result is that the actual EMR Record(s) will display. When multiple EMR records are found, they are stacked behind each other where the most recent appears in front. The user can page through the EMRs by pressing on an arrow key to page forward.

    b. Select the individual Physician. The result is the actual EMR records signed by that physician. When multiple EMR records are found, the records are stacked with the most recent record appears in front.

    c. Select individual Coder. The result is the actual codes and grouper results coded by that coder. Results are shown as stacks of documents which ban be paged through as described above.

    d. Select individual patient. The result is a list of all EMR records related to the patient's encounter during his/her episode of care.

3.5 Clinical Intelligence Dashboards & Statistical Methods

This specification defines the user selectable options for canned reports, dashboards and analytics typically found in Clinical Intelligence tools. To differentiate the higher value of Clinical Intelligence reports and analytics, I propose that canned reports and dashboards be divided into 3 categories of models: ***Basic***, ***Predictive*** and ***Advanced***. The tables in each category suggest the type of report, the statistical calculations and types of graphs. The basic reports include simple descriptive statistics. The Predictive and Advanced levels include advanced statistics and model-based analytics. The data scientists who build such reports and dashboards, could classify the reports into these 3 categories for improved user experience. The predictive and advanced reports might require additional input and statistical interpretation from the user. For example, the data scientist might offer not only the result of prediction or advanced analytics in a dashboard but also some statistical measures about accuracy of prediction, significance, generalizability of results and confidence level in the analytics produced. Some of these measures are discussed in Chapter 11.

3.6 Basic Models

The Basic models are essentially the OLAP Cube type reports. The user can drill down and roll-up on each slice of multi-dimensional data. These models compute simple but clever management metrics given the user's coding data. Note that medical service and medical unit are synonymous in this document. Unlike the traditional graphs, our graphs should indicate informative and statistically meaningful annotations. These annotations could consist of tick marks that indicate the 50%, 75% or 80% percentiles, one sigma, 2-sigma and 3-sigma variance from the mean, area under the curve, and a slide-bar that allows user interact with graphs so the user can select the percentiles and show results by highlighting that portion of the graph to convey additional information.

Model Category: Velocity of Data (Time-based)		
Model Name	**Model Description**	**Statistics**
Coding Lag	Duration from time doctor signs-off on a note to coder completes the code. Show results by: • Coder • Specialty • Physician • Actual coding lag variance from target coding lag • Procedure	Total Avg Min Max Std Dev 80% Percentile
Workflow Analyzer	Show the following: - The no. of notes received after the billing has been submitted - The time lapse and where the coding lag is below a threshold - Identify time lags in each step of the admit to billing process (productivity Analysis)	
Coding Queue	No. of cases waiting to be coded (in coding queue). Show results by: • Total no. in queue per day of week • Total no. in queue per hour of day • Total no. in queue by specialty per day of week • Rate of increase by specialty • Rate of increase by hour of day	Total Avg Min Max Std Dev 80% Percentile
Coder Takt time	The time spent by coders to code clinical notes. Show results by: • Time spent to code by specialty • Time spent to code by coder • Takt time by physician • Takt time by coder • Actual Takt time vs. Budgeted Takt time • Regression line of Takt time vs. medical diagnosis • Show or plot actual vs. budgeted reimbursement	Total Avg Min Max Std Dev 80% Percentile Regression line

LOS	Patient Length of Stay (LOS). Show results by: • Disease type (diagnosis type) • Physician • Nurse • Age • Gender • Insurance Payer • Specialty (or medical unit) • Trend line of LOS by Disease type • Regression line of LOS vs. disease type (to Identify outlier cases)	Total Avg Min Max Std Dev 80% Percentile Histogram to show trend line Regression line for Outlier identification
Discharge Rate	Data about rate of patient discharges. Show results by: • Surge rate of discharges by hour of day • Surge rate of discharges by day of week • Rate of discharge by nurse • Rate of discharge by specialty by day of week	Total Avg Min Max Std Dev 80% Percentile Histogram to show trend line

Model Category: Volume of Data		
Model Name	**Model Description**	**Statistics**
Code Rework	The volume of cases that need to be re-coded due to billing system rejection or insurance payer denial. Show results by: • No. of cases reworked by month & by week • Ratio of cases reworked divided by all cases • Time spent to rework cases by coder • No. of denial and reject cases by coder • No. of denial and reject cases by specialty • Dollar value of cases reworked by month & by week • No. of cases reworked by insurance payer	Total Avg Min Max Std Dev 80% Percentile
Error Cases	No. of incorrectly coded cases by different data slices. Show results by: • Specialty • Physician • Coder • Disease class • Show trend of errors by month & by week	Total Avg Min Max Std Dev 80% Percentile Histogram to show trend line
Claims Financials	Financial measures related to MS-DRG and coded claims. Show results by: • Dollar value of claims per insurance payer • Dollar value of claims by physician • Dollar value of claims by medical unit • Dollar value of claims by week	Total Avg Min Max Std Dev 80% Percentile Histogram to show

		trend line
Utilization Rates	Bed utilization and occupancy measures. Show results by: • Bed occupancy by day of the week • Bed occupancy trend line by day • Bed occupancy by diagnosis class • Bed turn-over rate • No. of surgeries per surgery room • No. of surgeries started on time • Utilization rate of surgery rooms as total and by room • Utilization rate of surgery rooms by day of week • How many hours was an OR room was utilized	Total Avg Min Max Std Dev 80% Percentile Histogram to show trend line

Model Category: Variety of Data		
Model Name	**Model Description**	**Statistics**
Re-admit Rate	Compute the number of re-admits to hospital within 30 days of a patient discharge date. Show results by: • No. of readmits per day • No. of readmits by disease class • No. of readmits by medical service (or medical unit)	Total Avg Min Max Std Dev 80% Percentile Histogram to show trend line
Hospital Acquired Complications	Count of hospital acquired complications over time. Calculate similar data to these shown below from the list of CMS published top 10 hospital acquired complications. Show results by: • No. of conditions after POA by day • No. of hospital acquired complications by physician • No. of hospital acquired complications by medical unit • No. of post-operative infection rates • Trend of post-operative infection rates by day • Trend of post-operative infection rates by medical unit • No. of cardiac arrests in hospital • Trend of cardiac arrests in hospital • No. of DVT & PE cases per week & per month • Trend of DVT & PE cases • No. of patients with Fall incidence • No. of patients with post-operative sepsis • No of patients with respiratory failure during their stay	Total Avg Min Max Std Dev 80% Percentile Histogram to show trend line

	• No. of patients with cases of UTI during their stay • No. of patients with hip fracture post-operation • No. of patients with cases of dehiscence post-operation • No. of patients with central venous line – catheter related infections	
MS-DRG	Calculations related to MS-DRG. Show results by: • MS-DRG by disease class • MS-DRG by medical unit • MS-DRG by physicians • MS-DRG by insurance • MS-DRG by LOS • MS-DRG by no. of patients • MS-DRG by day of the week • MS-DRG trends by day of the week	Total Avg Min Max Std Dev 80% Percentile Histogram to show trend line

3.7 Predictive Models

Predictive models demonstrate that given a real-time or regular (daily or hourly) batch data feeds Clinical Intelligence tools can generate predictive reports and analytics. Below is a summary of such reports:

Model Category: Velocity of Data (time-based metrics)		
Model Name	**Model Description**	**Statistics**
Discharge Prediction	By calculating the regression line of disease types, make predictions about the expected value of the following metrics. Show graphs of surge over the next 5-7 days on these metrics: • Expected discharge volume in the next 5-7 days by Specialty or medical service • Expected discharge volume in the next 5-7 days by disease class • Expected discharge volume in the next 5-7 days by Physician	Total Avg Regression line
Coding Queue Prediction	Predict No. of cases waiting to be coded (in coding queue) for the next 5-7 days. Show results by: • Expected total no. in queue per day of week • Total no. in queue per hour of day • Total no. in queue by specialty per day of week	Total Avg Regression line

Model Category: Variety of Data		
Model Name	**Model Description**	**Statistics**
Predict Re-admits	Predict the number of re-admits to hospital within 30 days of a patient discharge date. Show graph of surge for these metrics below. Show results by: • Which patients are likely to be re-admitted	Total Avg Min Max

	• Which medical service (or medical units) are likely to receive re-admits	Std Dev 80% Percentile Histogram to show trend line

3.8 Advanced Models

Advanced Models include statistical methods that bring new insights about the underlying relationships between the metrics and operational performance of the organization. These models consider relations between various demographic populations of patients, diseases and organization's performance.

Model Category: Variety of Data		
Model Name	**Model Description**	**Statistics**
Coding Correlation	Positive or negative statistical Correlation of coding metrics based on the following metrics: • Coding time lag • Coding Takt time • Disease class • Physician group or specialty • Medical unit (medical service) • Patient demographics (Age, Gender, etc)	Correlation Analysis ANOVA/MANOVA CHI Squared
ACO Correlations	Analytics useful to determine the cost of care by disease class for ACO management: • Cost calculations and variance (by RVU or dollars) of disease types • Cost calculations and variance (by RVU or dollars) by insurance payer	Frequency Diagram Correlation Analysis ANOVA/MANOVA CHI Squared
Patient population Mgt	Show patient counts of - Substitute meds cases (generic vs. brand meds) - Which patients need to be vaccinated among our patient population in the EMR database? - Flag patients who are due for follow ups	

3.9 Data Visualization Tools

This section presents various data visualization styles and examples to illustrate some of the possible clinical data visualization techniques. Several infographic and dashboard styles are presented. Frequently in building clinical analytics dashboards, data scientists combine these dashboards together to present what I call a "Mashboard", a mash-up of two or more dashboards. These sample graphs are illustrated by Pentaho[30]and Panopticon[31]. Additional dashboard styles can be found at Pentaho Community. The Pentaho community is a collaboration of users who share their dashboards with other community members[32].

Heat Maps

---

[30] www.Pentaho.com

[31] www.panopticon.com

[32] www.community.pentaho.com

A Heat Map is a set of square tiles that represent different values by different colors. Essentially, a Heat Map is a graphical representation of data where the values taken by a variable in a two-dimensional map are represented as colors. The color of the square represents a quantitative value relative to the other boxes in the Heat Map. They're ideal for visualizing large flat data volumes. Heatmaps and weather maps are closely related. They are used to graphically show changes in measurements across a certain area such as an anatomy at a given time. Some visualization tools ingest streaming data feeds in order to provide a real-time view of patient's physiological data. Just like the Heat map tool, the user can also hover over any item to bring up more detailed information on demand (Figure 3.5).

	Sun	Mon	Tue	Wed	Thu	Fri	Sat
0000	2.59	0.66	0.68	1.35	1.35	2.03	1.6
0100	1.39	0.7	0.95	1.22	1.08	1	2.12
0200	2.87	0.59	1.02	1.22	0.57	1.08	3
0300	0.99	0.25	0.5	0.48	0.5	0.99	1.7
0400	1.06	0.42	0.17	0.56	0.24	0.3	0.48
0500	0.32	0.23	0.39	0.22	0.47	0.47	0.44
0600	0.42	0.41	0.57	0.6	0.64	0.5	0.49
0700	0.38	1.29	0.77	0.86	1.42	1.14	1.22
0800	0.53	1.05	1.77	1.56	1.32	1.58	1.67
0900	0.62	2.04	2.97	1.45	2.96	1.92	2.32
1000	1.37	2.09	3.67	1.87	2.52	1.47	2.29
1100	0.98	3.27	1.6	3.32	2.89	2.09	1.27
1200	1.81	3.41	2.66	2.7	3.24	2.84	1.35
1300	2.38	1.79	2.15	1.91	1.64	1.43	2.49
1400	2.31	2.69	3.19	2.98	2.85	3.69	1.17
1500	1.44	1.46	1.44	3.46	1.55	3.55	2.35
1600	1.18	2.61	3.74	3.21	2.76	1.98	1.84
1700	1.52	3.45	1.4	1.99	1.79	3.33	2.1
1800	2.09	2.53	1.64	1.37	3.15	3.1	1.21
1900	2.67	1.2	1.44	2.04	2.58	1.16	2.34
2000	1.5	2.31	2.58	1.89	2.76	1.96	1.75
2100	0.81	1.7	1.97	1.76	0.99	3.16	1.92
2200	1.24	1.91	1.97	1.48	2.22	2.93	1.63
2300	1.69	1.55	1.74	1.29	2.01	1.97	3.87

Fig. 3.5 – Example of a Heat Map Graph

The Heat Map is very closely related to its more sophisticated cousin Treemap, except that a Heatmap represents each item in the database as an equally-sized square. A Treemap uses the size of the tile to represent a qualitative value, and location to represent hierarchical relationships. You can alter the color scale displayed in a Heatmap as needed in order to make it easier to spot outliers or reveal trends in the data sets you are examining.

Tree Maps

They display tree-structured data in an easy-to-understand, intuitive set of nested rectangles. Treemaps were invented by Professor Ben Shneiderman at the University of Maryland as a method to monitor and analyze disk space usage in his lab. In a Treemap, the size of a tile reflects its importance. The color conveys urgency. Typically shades of blue represent good news and shades of red represent bad news. Treemaps use people's innate ability to comprehend size, color and groupings very quickly – much faster than we can read and interpret reports, tables or diagrams (Figure 3.6).

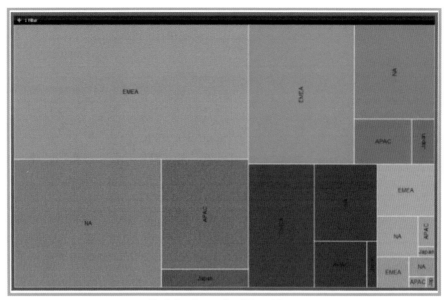

Fig 3.6 – Example of Tree Maps

Chord Diagrams

Chord diagram are used for exploring relationships between groups of entities. The thicker the chord size the higher or more significant the relationship is between the two entities. Chord diagrams are often used in Life Sciences for visualizing genomic data and other biological data visualization (Figure 3.7).

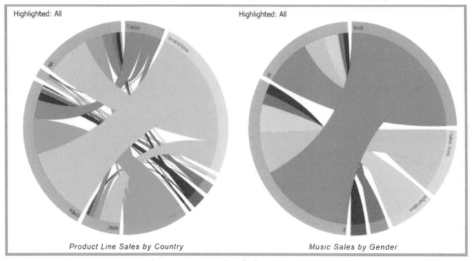

Fig. 3.7 – Example of Chord Diagrams

Parallel Coordinate charts

To visualize high dimensional data, parallel coordinate charts are suitable. This chart type enables users to visualize multiple attributes across many measures (Figure 3.8). Users can filter data of some or all measures to reduce dimensionality.

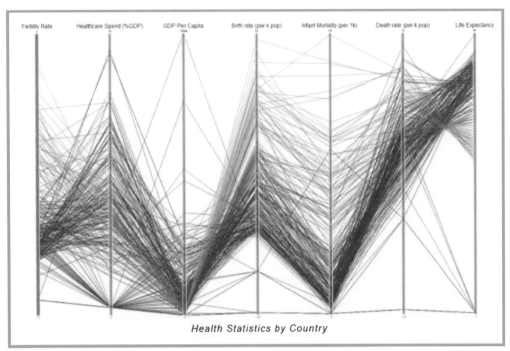

Fig. 3.8 – Example of Parallel Coordinate Charts

Index Charts

An index chart is a form of interactive line chart. It is helps visualize percentage changes for a set of time-series data based on an index point selected by user in the timeline. An example is shown in Figure 3.9 where the sales of several items for various months are compared to the month of July by relative percentage.

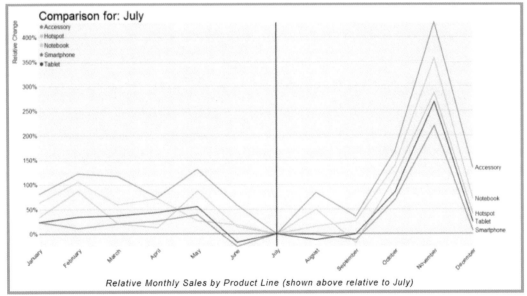

Fig. 3.9 – Example of Index Charts

Calendar chart

A form of heat map, Calendar chart helps visualize data values by their size and color arranged into days on a calendar. Days are arranged into columns by week, then grouped by month and years to form a heatmap arranged in a calendar format (Figure 3.10).

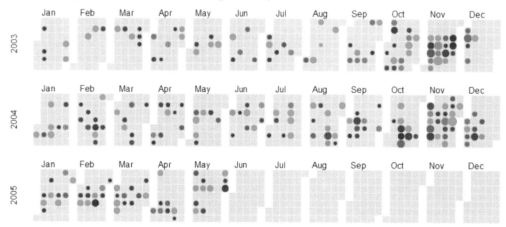

Figure 3.10 – Example of Calendar Chart

Heat Matrix Chart

The Heat Matrix is a form of Heat map data visualization. If the data items can be categorized into multiple groupings (for example, By Anatomy and By Disease Type), and you want to understand the correlation between these groupings the data can be presented in a Heat Matrix chart. It displays many different data items by representing the value for each item using colors. But unlike a Heatmap the Heat Matrix has a defined structure where two data attributes define each data item, thus producing a matrix. Within the Heat Matrix, each column and row represents a unique attribute, and the point where two items intersect represents the value or interaction of the two attributes.

Bar Graphs

Bar Graphs are one of the most popular and well-understood data visualizations used in BI Dashboards. Bar Graphs are especially useful when comparisons are critical to an understanding of the data. Bar Graphs — sometimes called Bar Charts — are easy to understand and are a great way to communicate important comparative information. Bar Graphs work especially well when comparing ten or fewer data items across a single quantitative variable. For displays including more than ten items, try using a Heat Map or Treemap instead. Bar Graph visualizations can be oriented horizontally or vertically in information displays, making them easier to incorporate into multi-visualization layouts. Some Bar Graph data visualizations[33] give you a number of different display options and are easy to work into almost any Executive Dashboard or other type of information display. Like Scatter Plots, Treemaps and other visualizations, Bar Graphs are designed to work with real-time streaming data sources as well as time series and static data. The simplest form of the Bar Graph is completely intuitive.

---

[33] For more examples, see data visualizations provided by Panopticon. (www.panopticon.com). The company was acquired by DataWatch in 2013. For additional and most up-to-date graphs also visit www.datawatch.com

The design of Bar Graph, like many information visualizations, Bar Graph emphasizes the data itself and eliminates unnecessary display items. For example, grid lines are designed to be background items that help make the Bar Graph easier to comprehend quickly without being a distraction. You can go further by enhancing the "data to ink ratio" by allowing Edward Tufte-syle grid line representations in which the grid is displayed by removing "ink" from the bars themselves.

Grouped Bar Graphs

The Grouped Bar Graph is an excellent way to show information about categorized groups of data in a single information visualization. Different colors make it obvious how items are related and provide an easy-to-read display.

Bar Graphs lets users plot historical data and predict future trends in seconds. They can slice and dice their data, drill down to view details, and compare several small or large time segments by creating new breakdowns on the fly. Simple, easy-to-read hover displays pop up when the cursor lingers over a single bar – or a selection of bars – in the Bar Graph, making it very easy to compare information about separate events in the timeline. Like in most visualizations, the Bar series can handle real-time streaming data feeds along with historical static data inputs.

Bullet Graphs

Bullet Graphs are easy to interpret and convey much more information than traditional tools using substantially less screen real estate. Bullet Graphs are the perfect element to add to Business Intelligence Dashboards to call attention to the status of Key Performance Indicators (KPI).

Bullet Graphs were developed by information visualization design expert Stephen Few. He created them to replace speedometers and gauges in executive BI Dashboards. They display information about a single quantitative measure like year-to-date revenue along with complementary measures to enrich the meaning of the featured parameter (See Figure 3.11). The linear design of the Bullet Graph gives it a very small footprint and makes them much easier to understand quickly than radial meters. As with most information visualizations, Bullet Graphs are ideal when they display real-time data — when they respond instantly to changes in the underlying data. You can feed them with any combination of historical data, calculated results and/or real-time data streams from message queues or other sources.

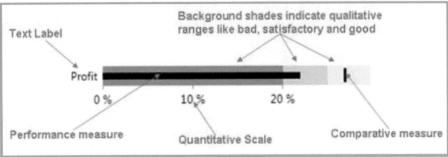

Fig 3.11 – Example of Bullet Graph

The Bullet Graph consists of these components:

- Text label
- A quantitative scale along a single linear axis
- The featured performance measure
- A comparative measure for reference purposes

Users find Bullet Graphs useful in a wide variety of use cases and are almost always included in information dashboards intended to provide quick overviews of Key Performance Indicators (KPIs). They take no time at all to understand and require no training. Their ability to highlight a single measure and simultaneously compare the status of a KPI with related factors make them invaluable in many deployments.

You can orient your Bullet Graphs horizontally or vertically and you can use several of them together to give users accurate information on several related KPIs at the same time. If you are designing an Executive BI Dashboard for Business Performance Management (BPM) or for monitoring and analyzing the performance of sales, marketing or other systems, Bullet Graphs will help you convey critical information to users effectively. They require no training and are easy to read at a glance.

Candlestick Graphs

Candlestick Graphs are a traditional financial visualization for display of time based price distributions. Specifically for each time slice, they display:

- Opening Price
- Highest Price
- Lowest Price
- Closing Price

Examples in healthcare include using Candlestick graphs to show patient's physiological data, blood pressure, temperature, heart rate and similar data that is typically gathered overtime from physiological monitors.

A Candlestick Graph is a style of Bar Graph used primarily to describe price movements of a security, derivative, or currency over time. It is a combination of a Line Chart and a Bar Graph, in that each bar represents the range of price movement over a given time interval. It is most often used in technical analysis of equity and currency price patterns.

Candlesticks are usually composed of the body (black or white), and an upper and a lower shadow (wick): the area between the open and the close is called the real body, price excursions above and below the real body are called shadows. Figure 3.12 shows an example Candlestick graph. The wick illustrates the highest and lowest traded prices of a security during the time interval represented. The body illustrates the opening and closing trades. If the security closed higher than it opened, the body is white or unfilled, with the opening price at the bottom of the body and the closing price at the top. If the security closed lower than it opened, the body is black, with the opening price at the top and the closing price at the bottom. A Candlestick need not have either a body or a wick.

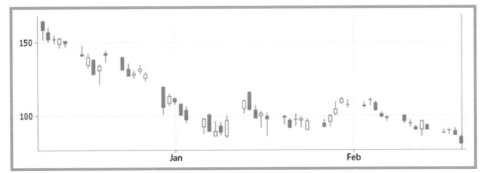

Fig. 3.12 – Example of Candlestick Graph

Traditionally, Candlestick graphs are used as a visual aid for decision making in stock, commodity, and option trading, but they have great applications in visualizing healthcare data. Candlesticks also show how prices are relative to the prior periods' prices, so one can tell by looking at one bar if the price action is higher or lower than the prior one. They can be colored for even better definition and visual analysis. Rather than using the open-high-low-close for a given time period (for example, 5 minutes, 1 hour, 1 day, 1 month), Candlesticks can also be constructed using the open-high-low-close of a specified volume range (for example, 1,000; 100,000; 1 million shares per Candlestick).

Dot Plot Graphs

The Dot Plot is an effective alternative to the Bar Graph data visualization in cases where the data contains groupings with similar values. Dot Plots do not use a zero baseline and are less cluttered than Bar Graphs, making them easier to interpret in many cases. In a financial dot plot graph shown in Figure 3.13, color indicates the One Day Change in price and the position of the dot on the horizontal axis represents the market cap for a database of equities. The stocks are grouped by country and a simple mouse move allows the user to aggregate up and down in the hierarchy.

In essence, Dot Plots are statistical charts consisting of groups of data points plotted on a simple scale. Typical uses for Dot Plots include continuous, quantitative, univariate data like comparisons of market capitalization for a large number of equities grouped by country.

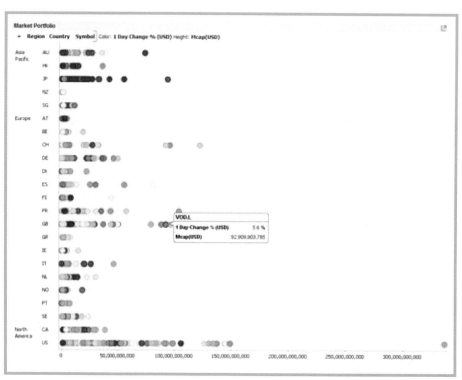

Fig. 3.13 – Example of Dot Plot Graph

Dot Plots are one of the simplest statistical data visualizations you can use and are good choices for small to moderately sized data sets. They are particularly useful for highlighting clusters and gaps, as well as outliers. The other major advantage of Dot Plots over Bar Graph or other visualizations is the conservation of numerical information.

Dot Plots are especially effective as a presentation tool to help people understand comparisons between grouped hierarchies of data. For example, sales reports that compare revenues by product line, store, region, department, and salesperson are a great place to use the Dot Plot. It's quite common to see such information displayed in tables. Unfortunately, this can make patterns in the data nearly impossible to see. Tables of data have their place, but in order to make good sense of them, you cannot simply read them as you can with a Dot Plot, you have to study them.

You can also use the Dot Plot information visualization to create Categorical Line Graphs. The X axis typically represents categorical periods like days or months rather than a specific time range. This form of the Dot Plot uses color to differentiate different categories of data and makes it easy to compare performance trends between categories.

One of the best characteristics of Dot Plots is that they help you present and compare fairly large amounts of data without using a lot of "ink on the page", in the words of information visualization expert Edward Tufte. They are compact and yet can convey a lot of useful, understandable information.

Horizontal Graphs

100

Horizon Graphs are an incredibly space effecent way to analyze and compare multiple time series data sets and compare trends. Horizon Graphs are a fantastic way to overview a large number of time series in a limited rectangular space. Horizon Graphs pack the information in a Line Graph in 1/6th the space using a smart pre-attentive color encoding algorithm. Users can scan huge amounts of data points across all relevant time series and immediately identify areas of concern that require closer scrutiny (Example in Figure 3.14).

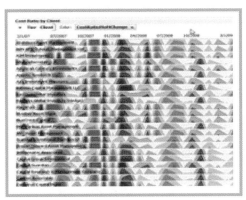

Fig. 3.14 – Example of Horizon Graph

Horizon Graphs were designed to make it easy to examine how a large number of items (clinical outcomes, prices, product sales, employee satisfaction, and other data) have changed through time. Horizon Graphs let you:

- Spot extraordinary behaviors and predominant patterns
- View each item independently from the others
- Make comparisons between items
- View changes with enough precision to determine if further examination is required

Building A "Mashboard"

You can compose your own "mashboard" by using Horizon Graphs in conjunction with Treemaps, Stack Graphs and other information visualizations to create an effective display of analytical dashboards. The Horizon Graph visualization is particularly useful when you need to see a large number of time series on a single screen. This makes it easy to compare trends and spot patterns that would be very difficult or impossible to see in a standard report. They work well in combination with Treemap, Heatmap and Scatter Plot visualizations in interactive analytical dashboards since they allow you to see your data from different perspectives. This data visualization displays quantitative values using a combination of length (like in a line graph, where the height of the curve represents the underlying value) and color (Figure 3.15). Users can read exact values from the visualization by hovering their cursor over specific points on the Graph.

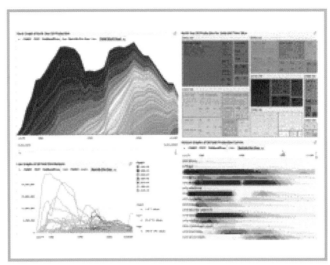

Fig. 3.15 – Example of a "Mashboard"

Line Graphs

Line Graphs are one of the most commonly used data visualizations. They are easy to understand and are a great way to communicate important comparative information about changes in data over time. They work especially well when comparing ten or fewer datasets. For larger numbers of data sets, try using Horizon Graph instead. The example in Figure 3.16 shows performance of 10 funds holding a specific equity. Each fund is represented by a different color.

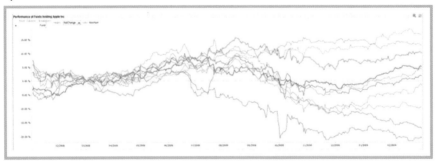

Fig. 3.16 – Example of Line Graph

The Y axis is based on percentage changes, making it easy to compare the relative performance of each sector. The Breakdown controls at the top of the graph allow users to select between Relative Performance and Absolute Performance views of the same data. Line Graph information visualizations give you many different options for setting up and displaying your data. You can configure them so that the X and Y axes relate to time or other quantitative factors. You can use color or line type to distinguish between the various datasets being displayed, which makes it easier to do comparisons.

Needle Graphs

Needle graphs are simple but highly functional way to visualize time series data. Needle Graphs display time based transactions or occurrence frequency, rather than time based trends. They are simply time based Bar Graphs where each bar is located at a particular time point on the axis. They work especially well when combined with a Line Graph. Needle Graphs are commonly used to display trading volume for a stock, commodity or other financial instrument, usually underneath a Line Graph correlated to price performance (Figure 3.17).

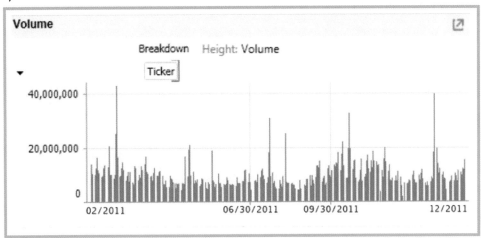

Fig. 3.17 – Example of Needle Graphs

Needle Graphs are particularly useful when combined with Line Graphs to compare trading volume with price performance for an equity or fixed income instrument. When the distribution of the data is more important than the trend, use a Needle Graph instead of a Line Graph. The example in Figure 3.18, shows a **Numeric Needle Graph** that displays price distributions for a product.

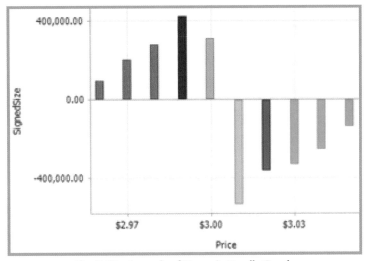

Fig. 3.18 – Example of Numeric Needle Graphs

Numeric Needle Graphs specialize in displaying price distributions. The X Axis is referenced to an arbitrary series of numbers instead of time. Like traditional Needle Graphs, they are simply a special kind of Bar Graph, but each bar in a Numeric Needle Graph is associated with a particular number in the numeric series used to generate the X Axis and their height is determined by their Y values. This allows gaps and clustering in price to be more accurately identified. They work especially well when combined with a Numeric Line Graph visualization[34].

Stacked Needle Graph

Stacked Needle Graphs allow you to see how constituents contribute to the total for time series data sets. Stacked Needle Graphs display time based transactions or occurrence frequency and are quite similar to the standard Needle Graph. However, Stacked Needle Graphs allow each transaction to be split into its components, which makes it easy to see contribution to the total across time (Example in Figure 3.19). Common uses for the Stacked Needle Graph include the split of transaction volume by venue or by direction (Buy versus Sell).

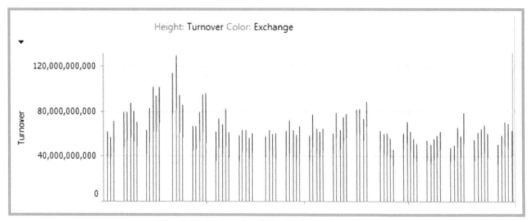

Fig. 3.19 – Example of Stacked Needle Graph

Pie Charts

The Pie Chart is perhaps the most popular data visualization in the world and is familiar to almost everyone. It displays fractions as "parts of the whole". Although popular, Pie Charts are not usually the most effective visualization technique for displaying data. For a small data set, the Bar Graph is more effective; for a large data set or a hierarchical data set, a Treemap is more useful.

Two distinct styles of Pie Charts

Pie Charts are popular visualization tools for Executive Dashboards and web-based presentations of data. A data visualization software can produce two different types of Pie Charts as illustrated in Figure 3.20. You can create a standard pie chart or a multi-level pie-chart as a Sunburst graph. A comparison of each type of pie chart with bar chart and Treemap are explained in Figure 3.20.

---

[34] www.panopticon.com/line-graph

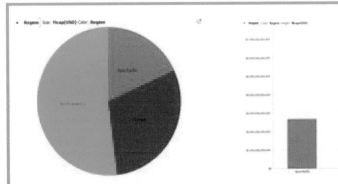

Standard Pie Chart — Each slice of the pie represents a numeric variable and its proportional relationship to the total. The color of each slice can represent a category or another numeric variable.

Compare this to a Bar Graph visualization using the same data. You do not need to use color to display an accurate and readable visualization and it's easy to see relative sizes as well as the absolute magnitude for each variable.

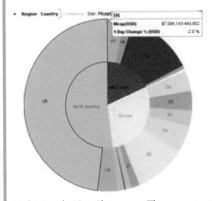

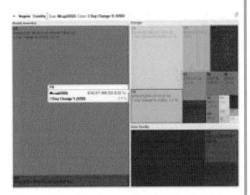

Multi-Level Pie Chart — These are also known as Sunbursts. They allow you to display a hierarchy within the data using multiple levels in the pie. You can modify the visible depth level to display only those levels in the hierarchy you want to see. You can also drill into a slice to see additional details about that specific subset of data.

Compare the Multi-Level Pie Chart to a standard Treemap data visualization, which allocates all of the available space to the visualization using rectangles rather than slices. Treemaps make more effective use of available space, enable more accurate comparisons and are an excellent way to display information about a large number of data points.

Fig. 3.20 – Two Styles of Pie Chart

Scatter Plots

Reports and standard table displays are hard and time-consuming to interpret, and aggregations of the data — which can make reports and tables easier to understand — can mask outliers, correlations and trends and make them difficult or impossible to see. Scatter Plots are an excellent information visualization to select when you are looking for positive and negative correlations, trends and outliers in large statistical databases. They are particularly useful in financial services applications.

Scatter Plot data visualizations are easy to set up and are highly customizable. You can configure your display in ways that will make the most sense to you, and users have all the tools they need to filter and manipulate the Scatter Plot to concentrate on the most relevant subsets in the data. Scatter Plots are a fairly sophisticated visualization and are best used to explore and discover new truths in your data. You can quickly identify anomalies and then take corrective action if needed while a problem is small — before it becomes unmanageable. Scatter plots are excellent graphs to spot correlations in data and expose outliers as shown in the example in Figure 3.21.

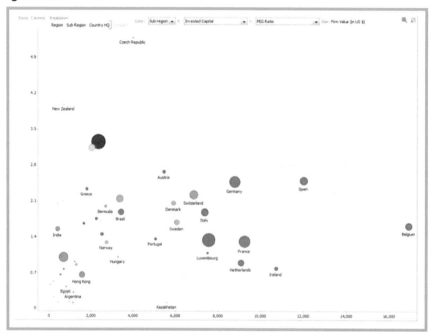

Fig. 3.21 – Example of Scatter Plot

Scatter Plots are particularly useful for finding outliers. In this example, you can see that Belgium has a very high PEG Ratio (X Axis) compared to its peers, especially when compared to the amount of Invested Capital (Y Axis).

Scatter Plots are a great companion to the other data visualizations— particularly the Treemap and Heatmap visualizations — and many analysts use them in multi-visualization displays. They can use the Scatter Plot to find interesting data points and then use other visualizations to look at the same data from different perspectives, or to present findings to their colleagues.

Geographic Scatter Plots

There are many instances when you must correlate changes in complex databases with physical locations. The Geographic Scatter Plot makes this easy and allows even the most non-technical users to explore and understand the information stored in their systems. Geographic Scatter Plots can sometimes reveal surprising and unexpected groupings that would be difficult to identify in traditional reports. They are also excellent presentation tools and can help convey important findings to the public or decision-makers (Figure 3.22).

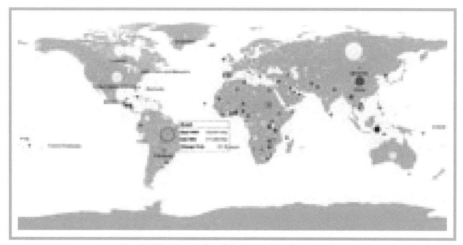

Fig. 3.22 – Example of Geographic Scatter Plots

Geographic Scatter Plots are ideal tools for presenting location-based data to non-technical users. Geographic Scatter Plot data visualizations are highly customizable. You can use any map image you like and define coordinate systems that match the resolution of your map. Hover displays automatically pop up when the cursor moves over a data point on the map to show detailed information. Some Geographic Scatter Plots also support all of the filtering and zooming tools you have come to expect in most data visualization software.

Spread Graph Visualizations

The Spread Graph displays the variance or spread between two time-based data series. It is a useful cousin of the Line Graph, Stack Graph and Horizon Graph time series data visualizations, but the Spread Graph is particularly useful for comparisons of two correlated series in order to identify important changes in the two series over time (Figure 3.23). You can combine Spread Graphs with Treemaps, Heatmaps or other similar visualizations to provide a more detailed view of the same data at a point in time selected from the Spread Graph.

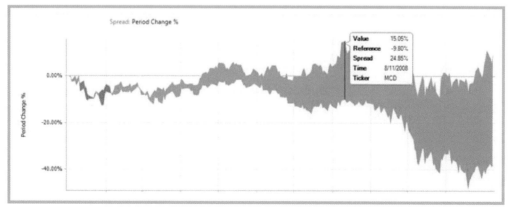

Fig. 3.23 – Example of Spread Graph

Spread Graphs are an excellent time series data visualization for dashboards that provide analytical views of equities, fixed income instruments - or any other data set - that must be compared to a benchmark. Financial services clients often use Spread Graphs in their analytical dashboards to:

- Compare a stock's price performance to a benchmark
- Compare the performance for two separate equities
- Compare a bond's yield to a benchmark rate or compare the yield of two bonds over time
- Compare the price performance of a mutual fund to a market index

Stack Graphs

Stack Graphs and Percentage Area Graphs help you analyze time series data. Stack Graphs are used to view components of totals. They let you visualize quantitative changes to several data sets over time, and you can see how each datapoint contributes to the total. This classic method for visualizing changes in a set of items lets you analyze the sum of the values as well as the individual items in a single chart.

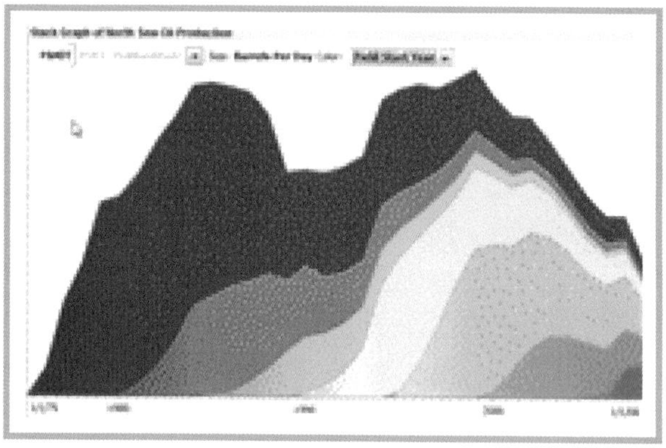

Fig. 3.24 – Example of Stack Graphs

Stack Graphs are a good choice when you have up to ten or eleven time series datasets to look at, especially for datasets that have a large number of positive datapoints. They are excellent information visualizations to use in conjunction with a Treemap, Heatmap or Scatter Plot tools since they provide different perspectives on the same set of data.

Percentage Area Graphs

Percentage Area Graphs are used to view relative contribution of constituents to the total. Percentage Area Graphs let you visualize quantitative changes to several datasets over time. You can see how each data point contributes to the total using these graphs (Example in Figure 3.25). The Percentage Area Graph form of the Stack Graph allows you to plot how the components contribute to the total (100%) in percentage terms. It is an excellent choice for charting time series data when you are interested in seeing the relative contributions for each data set in the series, regardless of the absolute total. This helps you see trends in how each component in the database has changed compared to the others which can easily be missed in a Stack Graph.

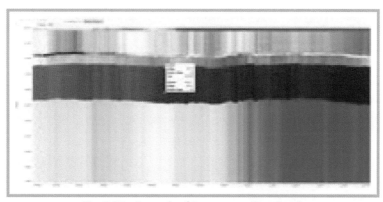

Fig. 3.25 – Example of Percentage Area Graph

Percentage Area Graphs let you visualize quantitative changes to several datasets over time, and you can see how each data point contributes to the total. However, instead of displaying absolute contributions as in the Stack Graph, the total is kept at 100% and each trace shows the relative portion of 100% that can be attributed to the total.

In a retail application, for example, Percentage Area Graphs are a great way to look at how sales of certain product lines are changing over time compared to all the other lines in the store. Applications include any instance where you need to be able to discern trends in market share, relative costs or relative profitability.

Surface Plots

Surface Plots are used to visualize trends in performance. Surface Plots display trending performance among three numeric variables. They are used to identify trends, and outliers within numeric surfaces. The Surface is made up of a series of points, where each point has an:

- X Position
- Y Position
- Color (which represents the Z Axis)

The Surface Plot can support data sets where the X and Y positions can both be regular and irregular in their distribution (Example in Figure 3.26). Additionally, the color scale can be continuous, or stepped to show a surface gradient. Surface plots are useful for visualizing matrices that are too large to display in numerical form and for graphing functions of two variables.

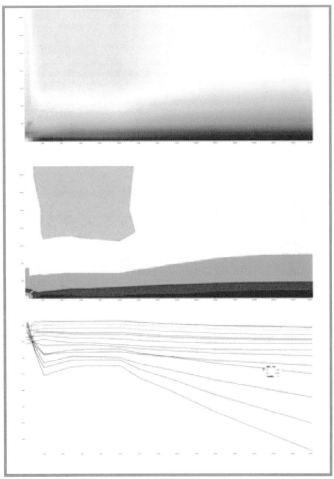

Fig. 3.26 – Example of Surface Plots

Complex Event Processing and Visualization of Results

Complex Event Processing (CEP) technology is rapidly becoming a standard tool in capital markets deployments, and soon will find its way in healthcare data visualization. Panopticon has developed a data visualization software that can handle direct real-time feeds from all popular CEP engines[35]. **With data coming in at more than 1000 events per second and nearly a quarter of stock market trading volume executed by software, Complex Event Processing (CEP) is rapidly becoming a key element in systems that support capital markets activities, but is likely to present a framework for healthcare and enter into healthcare industry as the number of sensors and monitors increase for inpatients and patient home care. The concepts of CEP and event visualization are likely to have a profound effect in healthcare.**

Visual analysis dashboards connected to CEP engines, databases storing historical time series data and real-time streaming sources provide users with the ability to filter, correlate and aggregate real-time event data

---

[35] Graphs were produced by Panopticon (www.panopticon.com) in 2012. The company was acquired by DataWatch in 2013. For additional and most up-to-date graphs also visit www.datawatch.com

in an extremely low latency environment (Figure 3.27 shows an example mashboard). The seamless integration of historical data with real-time events enables much more efficient trading since properly designed data visualizations reduce the time required to make well informed buy and sell decisions. In addition, detecting anomolous or potentially fraudulent behavior and gaming by individuals becomes much easier to accomplish is less time than ever before.

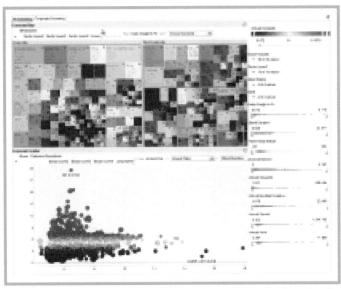

Fig. 3.27 – Example of a mashboard for Complex Event Processing Visualization

Tag Cloud (or Word) Cloud

Tag or Word clouds give a single visual of data frequency. Larger words (or tags) represent higher of frequency of search or occurrence value (such as sales or memberships). Below is the tag cloud of song sales sized by revenue and colored by downloads (Figure 3.28).

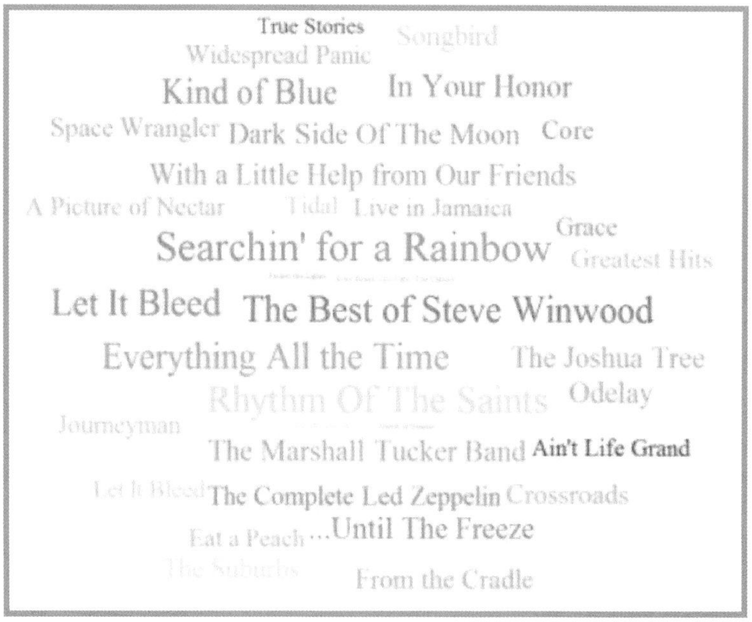

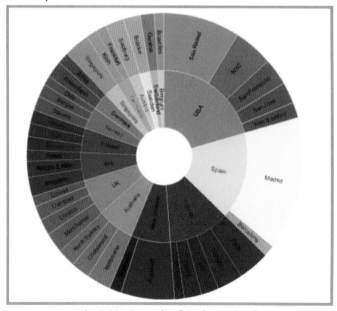

Fig. 3.28 – Example of Tag Cloud

Sunburst Graphs

A Sunburst graph might look like a multi-level pie chart. It shows data in a pie chart with constituent values corresponding to each slide of the pie. An sample Sunburst graph might look like the graph in Figure 3.29 that shows sales by regional hierarchy.

Fig. 3.29 - Example of Sunburst Graph

Zoom Chart

A Zoom chart is an interactive graph that allows user to zoom into a segment of the graph for more detail or enlarging that portion of the graph. Figure 3.30 shows an example of the Zoom chart.

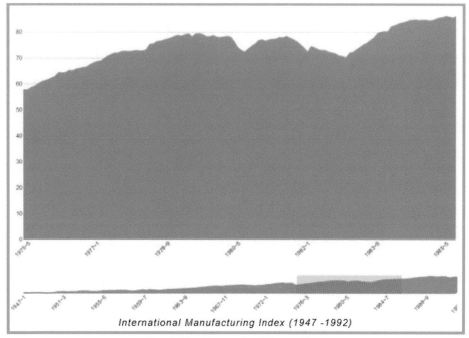

International Manufacturing Index (1947 -1992)

Fig. 3.30 – Example of Zoom Chart

Trellis Chart

Trellis charts provide a layout of smaller scatter plots in a grid with consistent scales. This style of graphs is called Trellis charts since they look similar to a garden trellis. Trellis charts are ideal for visualizing structure and patterns in complex data (Figure 3.31).

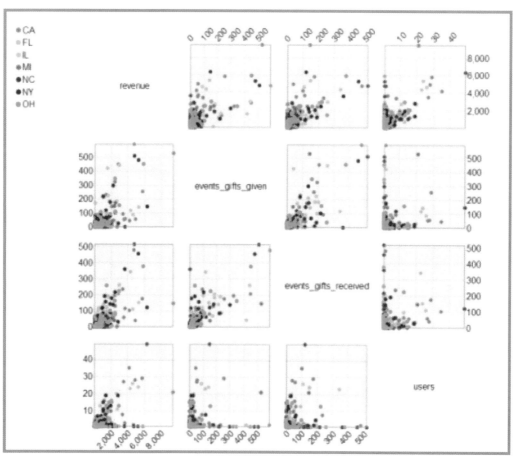

Fig. 3.31 – Example of Trellis Chart

Funnel Chart

This chart is similar to the stacked percent bar chart, except that it represents a diminishing volume through different stages from start of a process to the end of the process. Figure 3.32 shows a Funnel chart displays the reimbursement volume by the stage of patient length of stay (Courtesy, Pentaho Community)[36].

---

[36] Pentaho Community project site. http://wiki.pentaho.com/display/COM/Holiday+Visualizations. Last accessed: Jan 10, 2013.

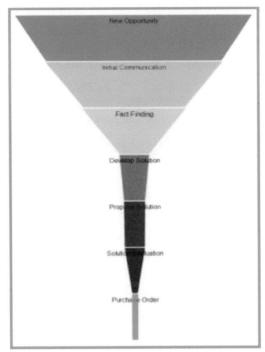

Fig. 3.32 – Example of Funnel Chart

Chapter 4

Clinical Prediction Rules

The following clinical prediction rules are commonly used in medicine to aid with clinical decision making. Clinical prediction rules are gaining popularity among physicians and have been advocated to enhance clinical judgment in diagnostic, therapeutic and prognostics.

CPRs are a field of medical research in which researchers attempt to identify rules for prognostics or diagnoses of disease by scoring a combination of medical signs, symptoms and other physiological and clinical findings (Jervis, McGinn 2008).

CPR scores are determined by researchers using algorithms that are predominantly based on linear regression or similar linear statistical methods. Despite advances with CPRs, it has been shown that physicians encounter lower accuracy and generalizability when they apply CPRs in their practice (Toll, Janssen, Vergouwe, Moons 2008). The key reasons cited for poor accuracy include differences from the initial patient population that the rule was developed and the current patient under treatment. This reflects on the fact that CPR rules are not extensible and adaptive enough to adjust to these differences. An adaptive method is needed to make more specific prediction tailored to a specific population of interest.

There are approximately 30 clinical prediction rules listed here but more are being validated and proposed every day through clinical research and analytics. These rules can be automated in clinical intelligence systems to bring a rich set of decision support and clinical alert to physicians and care providers. Clinical prediction rules (CPRs) can be combined into a mobile app as another compelling mobile tool for physicians. A clinical intelligence system can be developed to continuously extract specific data items from medical records, vital signs and lab results to provide alerts about specific patient conditions for each of these CPR rules in real time.

Clinical Prediction Rules	Description – Use case
CHADS2	Calculates patient risk of stroke with AFIB. C: Congestive Heart Failure. H: Hypertension. A: Age $\geq$ 75 yrs. D: Diabetes mellitus. S2: Prior Stroke or TIA or Thromboembolism.
CHADS2-VASc	Considers additional risk modifiers to CHADS2, such as: V: Vascular disease A: Age between 65-74 Sc: Sex category
APACHE II & APACHE III	Acute Physiology and Chronic Health Evaluation, measures severity of disease classification used for ICU scoring. It's appllied within 24 hours of patient admission to ICU.
CURB-65	A scoring method to predict mortality in community acquired pneumonia. C: Confusion of new onset U: Urea > 7 mmol/l R: Respiratory rate $\geq$ 30 breaths per min B: Blood pressure < 90 mmHg systolic or diastolic blood pressure

	≤ 60 mmHg
Ranson Criteria	Used for predicting the severity of acute pancreatitis. It has two algorithms to predict at admission and within 48 hours of admissino. It uses the following measure to compute the predictive score at admission (details for 48 hour algorithm will be added later): Age > 55 years White blood cell count > 16,000 cells/mm^3 Blood glucose > 10 mmol/L Serum AST > 250 IU/L Serum LDH > 350 IU/L
MELD	Model for End-stage Liver Disease, is a scoring prediction model to assess severity of chronic liver disease. Was previously used to predict death within 3 months of patients undergoing transjugular intrahepatic protosystemic shunt (TIPS) procedure and is now being used for prognosis of patients with liver transplant procedures. It's now being widely used by many organizations. MELD = 3.78 *[(Ln serum bilirubin (mg/dL)] + 11.2* [(Ln INR] + 9.57* [Ln serum creatinine (mg/dL)] +6.43. The interpretation of MELD score is dependent on another formula based on patient age.
PORT Score or PSI (Pneumonia Severity Index)	Predicts the probability of morbidity and mortality among patients with community acquired pneumonia. It classifies pneumonia patients into Risk Class I, II or III. When used for mortality prediction, it's the same as CURB-65.
Wells Score	A prediction rule used for scoring two complications: DVT probability scoring for diagnosing deep vein thrombosis, and for Pulmonary embolism (PE) probability scoring for diagnosing PE.
Ottawa Ankle Rules	Set of criteria used to determine whether X-Ray is appropriate for patients with ankle pain.
Pittsburg Knee Rules	Set of criteria used to determine whether x-Ray is justified to assess a fracture in patients with knee injury.
Physiotherapy Rules	A large number of rules have been developed for physiotherapy practice that helps with physical examinations and defines which therapeutic routines are appropriate given patient's head, neck, extremities, upper and lower back conditions.
MEDS Score	Mortality in Emergency Department Sepsis score is a prediction rule to predict death and stratification risk of patients with infection to predict their mortality rate.
Renal Artery Stenosis	A prediction rule to select patients for renal angiography among patients with renal artery stenosis (narrowing of blood vessels in kidney)
The Rule of 7's	A set of clinical prediction rules to predict meningitis (Lyme Meningitis vs. aseptic Meningitis) among children by considering situation when 3 factors are met such as: Headache < 7 days Cerebrospinal Fluid (CSF) mononuclear cells < 70% Absence of seventh or other cranial nerve palsy.
Diagnosis of Acute Meningitis in Adults	Rule set for diagnosis of acute meningitis among adults as published by Journal of General Internal Medicine

Feasibility study of predictive models based on artificial neural networks to assist physicians as alternate scoring method to CPRs is a worthwhile research because it provides deeper clinical intelligence about the patients' clinical status and diagnosis. CPRs are a branch of evidence-based medicine. Examples include Wells score[37], Ottawa ankle rules[38], Ranson criteria[39] and Apache II[40]. It has been posited (Laupacis, Sekar, Stiell 1997) that the purpose of prediction rules is to "suggest a diagnostic or therapeutic course of action." Almost all prediction rules in use today provide diagnostic or prognostic probabilities, typically by using a score or risk-stratification algorithm.

Prognostics methods using Artificial Neural Networks (ANN) promise to deliver new insights into patient health status that provide more effective medical treatment during the patient hospital stay. Using predictive models as a standard of care promises to improve patient care and diagnostic quality by providing advanced knowledge of patients' impending health status. These topics are covered in Part II.

---

[37] Wells score is a clinical prediction rule developed by Wells that predicts a patient's probability of acquiring pulmonary embolism.

[38] Ottawa ankle rules are guidelines that doctors in deciding if a patient who presents with foot or ankle pain should be offered X-rays to diagnose a possible bone fracture.

[39] Developed in 1974, Ranson rule is a clinical prediction rule for predicting acute pancreatitis.

[40] APACHE II (Acute Physiology and Chronic Health Evaluation II) is one of several ICU scoring systems that offer severity of disease classification score, an integer between 0 to 71 to patients admitted to Intensive Care Unit (ICU).

PART II

Clinical Prognostics and Prediction

Chapter 5. Clinical Intelligence Methods

Using machine learning algorithms researchers can detect patterns in data, perform classification of patient population, and cluster data by various attributes. The algorithms used in this analysis include various neural networks methods, Principal Component Analysis (PCA), Support Vector Machines, supervised and unsupervised learning methods such as k-means clustering, logistic regression, decision tree, and support vector machines.

Other methods include graphical reasoning, a form of case-based reasoning. These techniques enable the researcher to identify a specific clinical case and then search through the clinical data and identify other cases that match the specific clinical case.

Other techniques start by marking key events in the specific clinical case as a Graph of Planned States (GOPS). The search through medical records attempts to identify all cases that match or deviate from the planned graph. This technique is used to identify those patient care episodes that deviated from the specified plan of care. The actual care events are marked as the Graph of Observed States (GOOS).   Researchers can identify all other cases that match the GOPS graph and those cases that should but don't match the GOPS. Figure 5.1 shows the graph containing key events of administering appropriate antibiotics to patients post-surgery (on the left) and the abstracted GOPS graph on the right.

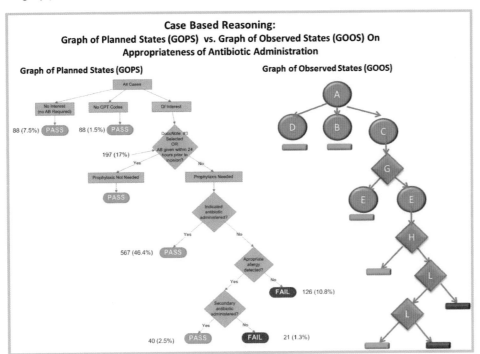

Fig. 5.1. Example of Case Based Reasoning Graph to Extract Antibiotic administration Deviations

5.2 Clinical & Predictive Analytics

Predictive Analytics is intended to provide insight into future events. It includes methods that produce predictions using supervised and unsupervised learning. Some of the methods include neural networks, PCA and

Bayesian Network algorithms. Predictions require the user to select the predictive variables and the dependent variables from the prediction screen.

A number of algorithms are available in this category that provide a rich set of analytics functionality such as Logistic Regression, Naive Bayes, Decision trees and Random forest, regression trees, linear and non-linear regression, Time Series ARIMA[41], ARTXp, and Mahout analytics (Collaborative Filtering, Clustering, Categorization). Additional advanced statistical analysis tools are often used, such as multivariate logistic regression, Kalman filtering, Association rules, LASSO and Ridge regression, Conditional Random Fields (CRF) methods, and Cox Proportional Hazard models to support text extractions. A brief mathematical overview of these techniques appears in the next section.

5.2 Analytics Summary

The following section is a peek into a common list of analytic algorithms in healthcare diagnosis, research and prediction.

- Linear Regression – The goal of linear regression is to find a linear equation that best fits a set of data. A data point may consist of multiple dependent variables. For example, when there are two dependent variables, the best fit equation is a plane through the observed dependent data values. For example, a user might be interested in computing the regression graph for patient Length of Stay (LOS) using three independent variables, patient AGE, Systolic and Diastolyc patient Blood Pressure (BP).

- Kalman Filtering – This technique is used to predict the future value of certain dependent variable over time. It works by using the most recent values of a variable and adjust the prediction by minimizing error between the predicted and observed result. The result is fed back into the model to make the next prediction at a lower error value. It can be used to predict short term values of patient's blood pressure, temperature and other physiological measurements if adequate historical data can be accumulated.

- LASSO – A regularized version of least squares method is the Least Absolute Shrinkage and Selection Operator (LASSO) method. LASSO is preferred for computing compressed sensing, a technique in signal processing to acquire and reconstruct a signal by solving the undetermined linear systems thus the entire signal can be reconstructed from a relatively few measurements. Its application in healthcare include improving MRI and CT image processing, as well as pattern recognition in patient image data.

- Multivariate Logistic Regression – The Multivariate logistic regression is a form of regression analysis used for predicting the result of a categorical dependent variable subject to one or more predictor variables. Examples of categorical variable in healthcare can be gender (MALE, FEMALE). This is a binomial or binary logistic regression since the outcome can have only two possible values. Other categories may have been created from continuous data. For example, weight can be categorized as LOW, MED and HIGH based on certain thresholds. Logistic Regression is used extensively in healthcare and medical research. One of the widely used methods to predict mortality in injured patients called Trauma and Injury Severity Score (TRISS) is an example[42].

---

[41] Auto Regressive Integrated Moving Average.

[42] Boyd CR, Tolson MA, Copes WS. Evaluating trauma care: the TRISS method. Trauma Score and the Injury Severity Score. J Trauma. 1987 Apr;27(4):370-8. URL: http://www.ncbi.nlm.nih.gov/pubmed/3106646

- Association rules – A technique used in machine learning to develop association rules between texts when data mining. In clinical domain, this technique discovers associations between clinical terms in EMR documents. For example, a rule {beta blocker, Adenosine} => {Rapid Heart Rhythm} would indicate that if a patient presents with terms beta blocker and Adenosine medications, there are likely to have been treated for SVT (Supraventricular tachycardia), a rapid heart rhythm condition.

- Ridge Regression – Also referred to as Tikhonov regularization, is a form of least squares method. It has been used in medical research to predict patient diseases and their stage of disease growth. For example, it has been used to predict which stage of disease patients are going to present in the next few months or predict cancer recurrence in patients.

- Decision trees and Random forest – Decision tree and its cousin influence diagrams are similar graphical methods of calculating the expected values (or expected utility) of competing alternative decisions. Its application in medicine is in medical diagnosis and decision analysis.

- Time series ARIMA – Autoregressive-Integrated-Moving-Average models are used to predict the next value in a given time series dataset. Given a time series data set, the ARMA model uses two parts, an autoregressive (AR) component and a moving average (MA) component to predict the future values in the series. Their application in healthcare has been proven in medical emergency such that it can detect abnormally high visit rates related to a particular disease that may be an early signal of an outbreak, epidemic or bioterrorist attack.

- ARTXp – The autoregressive Tree with Cross Connect model is similar to ARIMA except that it uses a decision tree algorithm to predict the next value in periodic time series data. If the user is interested in finding only the next value in a recurring time series data set, ARTXp is recommended.

- CRF methods - Conditional Random Fields are excellent for pattern recognition and machine learning since they take context into account. Often used for parsing sequential data, they can predict the next word in a sequence of phrases. In medical research, CRF methods which are a supervised machine learning technique have been used to train the model to identify negation successfully.

- Cox Proportional Hazard models – Proportional hazard models are a form of survival models. These models calculate the time that passes before some event occurs to one or more covariates that are associated with the outcome.

- Naïve Bayes method – The goal of Naïve Bayes method is to classify data using simple probabilistic Bayes' theorem with strong (naïve) independence assumptions. This method is popular among physicians for diagnosis and prediction because it is simple but accurate and can explain how it arrived at a classification. NB methods have been used in medical research to predict and diagnose a number of diseases ranging from cancers to hepatitis and liver disorders.

- ANOVA/MANOVA – Analysis of variance and multivariate analysis of variance measure how congruent or incongruent the variance changes in variables are with each other. These tools have been used to determine the impact of drugs on controlling disease symptoms.

- Principal Component Analysis – The PCA method are closely related to factor analysis. They're excellent for classification & prediction of independent variables and their contribution to the outcome (dependent variable). It's a method that translates correlated variables into uncorrelated variables. They are used in medical research for identify the key principle factors that affect or classify a patient's disease. They've been used in genetics to identify the internal structure of a given genetic data set and diseases, as well as identify which datasets are similar.

5.3 Probabilities and Odds Ratio

In probability, when we measure the chance that an event occurs, we divide the number of occurrence by the total number of opportunities for the event to occur. For example, the probability to get a 6 when we roll a die is 1/6. The probability that two events occur simultaneously is multiplicative. So the probability that a player gets a double 6 when rolling two dices is 1/6*1/6 = 1/36.

Odds are typically expressed as a ratio, rather than a fraction; probability is expressed as a fraction. Probability describes the fraction of time that you can expect an event to occur; Odds describe the ratio of time that the event occurs to the time that it does not. Odds of rolling 6 are once for every 5 times that you roll something else. The odds can be from 0:1 when something never happens, to 1:0 when something always happens. Odds of 1:1 are fifty-fifty, equally likely to occur or not, which corresponds to 50% probability. A player who rolls the same dice can expect to see 6 with the odds of 1 to 5. In other words, if I bet $1 to your $5 that I will roll a 6, the bets will be even in the long run.

Results of Logistic Regression are Clinical Intelligence is typically expressed in odds ratios.

Additive Interaction of Odds Ratio

Often we're interested in the interaction of risk factors, the extent to which the joint effect of two risk factors on disease differs from the independent effects of each of the factors (Kalilani, Atashili, 2006). The joint effect is the effect of the presence of both factors on disease and the independent effect is the effect of each factor in the absence of the other factor. In terms of their causal effects on the incidence of a disease, two risk factors may act independently or interact thereby augmenting (in case of synergism) or reducing (in case of antagonism) the effect of one another. Researchers consider two distinct types of interaction, biological interaction and statistical interaction. Statistical interaction is a model-dependent construct. It is considered to be present on a multiplicative scale when the joint effect of risk factors differs from the product of the effects of the individual factors. Statistical interaction is present on the additive scale when the joint effect of risk factors differs from the sum of the effects of the individual factors.

Biological interaction infers causality and refers to the interdependent action of two or more factors to produce or prevent certain effect. The combined interaction is sometimes regarded as spurious effects of these independent variables. The biological interaction is very difficult to measure and difficult to infer. We know that correlation does not infer causality. In order to show two or more variables have combined effect, study of their casual diagrams is needed.

5.3 Clinical Prognostics & Prediction

As we climb the Clinical Intelligence Maturity Model, we find prediction and clinical decision support at the higher levels of this framework. This section offers three key ideas related to classification, decision support and prediction. First, it develops a control system treatment of medical prognostics and predictive models. The control system development of prognostics combines feed-forward and feedback control mechanisms to create a framework for medical prognostics. This framework introduces a rules-based prognostics engine that uses ANN algorithms to identify patients who develop a particular disease or medical complication.

Second, it provides a generalized committee of models framework to predict the patient's medical condition and predict any medical complication from large data sets. The model also provides the strength (or the impact level) of all contributing clinical data to that prediction. The methodology proposes using a multi-algorithm prognostics framework to enhance the accuracy of prediction using four ANN models. The framework introduces a supervisory program, called an oracle[43] to select the most appropriate ensemble of models that best meet the practitioner's desired prediction accuracy.

Third, it demonstrates the viability and feasibility of using ANN methods as predictive models in this framework. As part of a case study and for illustration this part explores building, training and validating four ANN models to predict medical complications from data acquired from patients' hospital stay to predict Deep Vein Thrombosis/Pulmonary Embolism (DVT/PE)[44].

The aim of all three ideas is to improve the physician's ability to make predictive decisions from a vast array of data in order to be proactive and apply preventative medical interventions before complications occur.

5.4 Motivation

Predicting medical conditions for patients during their hospital stay is regarded as one of the most challenging and rewarding undertakings for physicians when such predictions are timely and informative enough for medical intervention. During their course of care, patients frequently experience escalating health problems that lead to further medical complications. These complications, mostly regarded as preventable (Maguire 2007), cause severe pains, injuries, disabilities and even death among patients. Several studies have suggested that complications are common with estimates of frequency ranging from 40% to 95% (Davenport, Dennis, Wellwood, Warlow 2006), and some relate poor outcomes to such complications (Johnston, Lyden, Hanson, Feasby, et al 1999). Prediction and diagnosis of escalating medical conditions has been a province of Clinical Prediction Rules (CPRs).

In another research front, prediction has been a topic of study by engineers. To apply an engineering approach to prediction, interest in Prognostics and Health management (PHM) field has been growing (Pecht 2008). PHM is a discipline focused on predicting the time at which a component in a system will no longer perform as intended. When applied to medical prediction, PHM predicts when a physiological organ will fail or when a disease will occur. PHM is a relatively new field that promises to help medical prognostics (Ghavami, Kapur 2011). Among adaptive mathematical methods used for prognostics, Artificial Neural Networks (ANNs) have become popular in the last two decades as powerful prediction tools. ANNs owe their popularity to their ability to model non-linear relationships, handle adaptive learning, pattern recognition and classification – features that can be helpful in building medical predictive models.

Despite advances with Clinical Prediction Rules (CPRs), it has been shown that physicians encounter lower accuracy and generalizability when they apply CPRs in their practice (Toll, Janssen, Vergouwe, Moons

---

[43] In the historical and mythical context of Greek culture, an oracle was a mythical person who foretold the future.
[44] DVT/PE, is a condition caused by blockage of patient lung vessels by blood clots that initially form in patient's legs. DVT/PE leads to severe pain, loss of lung function and even death.

2008). The reasons for poor accuracy are generally attributed to differences between the patient data under treatment and the initial population that the rule was developed. These differences are due to geography (the region or site) differences, domain differences (age, sex or clinical specialty) and temporal differences (rules become less accurate "over time"). Physicians often find prediction quite challenging due to this difficulty plus four additional challenges: 1) not all input data required by the CPR may be available; 2) not knowing when a particular CPR rule is applicable, 3) A CPR does not exist, or the CPR score is not definitive, and 4) The research is contradictory or inconclusive.

The rise in sensor technology now affords us with more accurate and frequent data collection methods. Frequency of lab test results, diagnostic tests and even the genomics data that's becoming easier to obtain combined with advances in computer storage systems afford large sums of data accumulation per patient. This gives rise to a "big data problem" in medicine that provides both a challenge and opportunity. The challenge is that the data volumes are vast and are getting larger, so big that they exceed human cognition's limits for analysis. The opportunity is that new and diverse analytical tools can be applied to assist physicians in diagnosis and even prediction.

Yet the tools necessary to analyze such big data are still not fully standardized and remain exclusive to researchers. Modern technology has made it possible for medicine to collect a vast amount of physiological data from patients during their course of treatment. Prior research has focused primarily on using this data for diagnosis, based on prior clinical evidence. But development of analytical tools for predicting medical conditions using real-time physiological data has been under explored. Early detection of medical complications and adverse conditions allow physicians to apply appropriate interventions that prevent adverse outcomes. Even though predictive and preventative medical interventions are preferred over the reactive methods, the predictive Clinical Intelligence has not found its rightful place in the gold standard of medical practice. Further research and development are necessary to advance predictive Clinical Intelligence into robust, practical and every day standard medical tools.

Medical science is grounded in scientific evidence, prior research, experiments and studies that have produced a body of medical knowledge based on generalizations and meta-analysis of research data. Such generalizations explain the causal relationships between risk factors, diseases and diagnosis. There are however gray areas in medical prognostics because many health treatment and screening decisions have no single 'best' choice and because there is scientific uncertainty or the clinical evidence is insufficient (O'Connor, Bennett, Stacey, et al. 2009). In many areas of medical science, the causal relationships are still incompletely understood and controversial. There are environmental, situational, cultural and unique factors that provide specific clinical data about a disease or groups of patients. Although this data is inadequate for making scientific generalizations and clinical evidence, it can provide valuable information to make assessments of individual's health status.

Therefore, a computational model that can adapt to specific domains, patient demographics and geographies is desirable and useful in providing clinical predictions using available physiological data from patients under treatment. Since Artificial Neural Networks are able to model non-linear data relationships and to adapt to new data sets, they are promising tools for this computation model.

However, clinical prediction models such as the model developed in this book become more feasible for physicians to use for data mining and extracting relevant information to predict where the patient's health is headed.

A large volume of literature concerning mathematical models to predict biological and medical conditions has been published. But only a few of such works in predictive mathematical tools have found their way into mainstream clinical applications and medical practice. Several reasons are cited for the low adoption of predictive tools: either important biological processes were unrecognized or crucial parameters were not known, or that the mathematical intricacies of predictive models were not understood (Swierniak, Kimmel, Smieja 2009). When such parametric or evidence-based knowledge are not available, prognostics framework described in this framework can be crucial to making clinical decisions.

Generally, most of the predictive methods previously proposed are based on a single model. The concept of ensemble of models (also known as committee of models) has received considerable attention in recent years. The main idea of ensemble of models is to combine the outputs of several models into a single predictor. While the concept of committee models has been used in other domains of research in the past, only a few (Ghavami, Kapur 2011) have investigated the viability of committee models in the clinical domain, trained on clinical data for medical prediction.

5.5 Framework for Advanced Clinical Intelligence

Despite the rise in volume, velocity and variety of clinical data, little attention has been paid to developing a framework for prediction of patient health status using prognostic methods on these large data sets. This framework develops and explores a multi-model prognostics framework for prediction and demonstrates its feasibility as a systemic prognostics method to predict patient health status.

The first concept in this framework is the introduction of control system treatment of prognostics and feed-forward model of clinical prediction. Another chapter focuses on the evaluation of feasibility and viability of using various algorithms (Support Vector Machines, Neural Networks, Bayesian Nets) as a medical prognostics analytic methods. Among feasibility elements, accuracy and generalizability of ANN models will be examined.

The second concept in the framework is the comparison of multiple analytics algorithms using the same case study. The intent of using multiple analytical models is to account for diversity in clinical data types. Some analytical models are more accurate and perform better on certain class of data than others. No single algorithm can be ideal for different types or volume of clinical data. Using four independent analytical models ensures that results from a sampling of various models are considered. Finally, a framework for comparison of the four models on accuracy characteristics is provided. This framework along with a supervisory oracle program that selects the most accurate algorithm or ensemble of algorithms enhances the model's accuracy.

The aim of this chapter is to improve the physician's ability to make proactive and preventative medical interventions, namely decisions, to prevent future complications and derive knowledge necessary for evidence-based medicine in advance.

There are five critical factors that define applicability, viability and feasibility of using analytical models as a prognostics tool. These factors fashioned after Smye and Clayton's work on mathematical models in medicine can be defined by the following criteria (Smye, Clayton 2002):

1. Accuracy: Accuracy of prediction
2. Well-posedness: Stability & immunity to small perturbations of input data

3. Utility: Applicability, practicality and usability in the medical workflow
4. Adaptability: Ability to handle new evidence, i.e. new data values and data types
5. Economy: Cost of computation and timeliness of prediction

To explore the above critical factors in real case study, a prognostics model using four different types of analytics algorithm are compared in the following chapters. The prediction accuracy of each model is compared to the actual clinical outcomes from prior retrospective patient cases. Analysis about accuracy includes measurements such as calibration (agreement between predicted probability and observed outcome frequencies), discrimination (ability to distinguish between patients with and without the disease), sensitivity (true positive rate, or proportion of patients who are correctly diagnosed as having the disease), specificity (true negative rate, the proportion of healthy patients who are correctly diagnosed with negative result), likelihood ratio (LR, the likelihood that a given test result would be expected in a patient with the disease compared to the likelihood that the same result would be expected without the disease) and receiver operating characteristic (ROC, a plot of true positive rate vs. false positive rate, namely a plot of sensitivity vs. one minus the specificity) curves (CEBM 2012).

Model validity (do the model's results match the reality), accuracy (the closeness of results to the quantity's actual value) and precision (the degree in which repeated measurements under unchanged conditions produce the same result) are compared among the four analytical models using clinical outcomes of prior patient data obtained from retrospective studies. But, clinical field validation and impact analysis on prospective cases are important topics but outside the scope of this book. Those interested in field validation can find many texts in clinical trial and meta-analysis that address these topics more fully.

Most medical predictive models provide crude and general predictions based on risk factors over a long time horizon that range from several months to several years in the future. A major contribution of this book is the development of a neural network predictive model with a trainable rule-based engine that provides continuous predictions of patient health status using real time patient physiological data. The goal of the prognostic model is to offer predictions for a patient's health status over a short term time horizon. In other words predict adverse or abnormal conditions in a time period ranging from a few seconds to several hours from any given the current time.

5.6 Significance of Predictive Clinical Analytics

The Evidence-based Medicine Working Group (McGinn, Guyatt, Wyer, Naylor, Stiell, et al. 2000) has proposed that prediction rules can "change clinical behavior and reduce unnecessary costs while maintaining quality of care and patient satisfaction".

Physicians struggle to incorporate the best evidence into their daily work. However, the vastness of clinical data and diverse patient situations make it difficult for physicians to remember all applicable CPRs and compute them correctly at any given moment. Developing a prognostics model that can learn and adapt to specific clinical environments and patient population is highly desirable.

The application of Prognostics Health Management (PHM) to human physiological measurement data promises to conceptually deliver several benefits such as:

1. By continuously and iteratively assessing the physiological and biological input data provide prediction and advanced warning of medical complications.

2. A localized prediction tool that incorporates nuances of local population and clinical environment.

3. Ability to analyze large data sets and provide trained models for prediction.

Continuous and periodic monitoring of the individual's physiological systems involves collecting data from historical patient physiological data ranging from circulatory to respiratory and immune systems. The PHM method used in this book considers prognostic models built upon prior data from retrospective cases in order to make predictions about a new patient.

The following section reviews the prior research and published literature in these areas.

5.7 Prior Research & Literature Review

In order to cover relevant prior research literature critical to this framework, studies from a confluence of three areas are examined. These areas are: Clinical Prediction Rules, Prognostics and Health Management, and an overview of clinical statistical methods including logistic regression, decision trees, Case-based reasoning (CBR). In addition, relevant prior research in Prognostics, Artificial Neural Networks and model validation are covered. A summary of prior research limitations are also presented. The diagram below is the epistemology of CPR research and literature review (Figure 5.2):

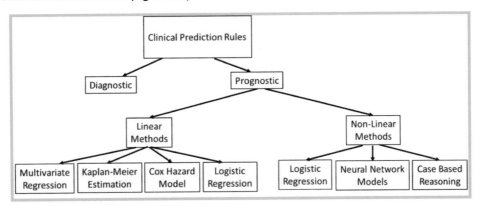

Fig. 5.2 - Epistemology of prior Clinical Prediction Rule methods

Modern healthcare strives to improve patient care and extend lifetime by using state of the art techniques and equipment. Among techniques available, predictive and preventive approaches are highly desired since they can reduce medical complications and reduce healthcare costs. As the sophistication and availability of medical devices and sensors have risen in recent years, more data is being collected that can aid in patient prognostics.

Similarly, sensors and data acquisition components have become smaller and cheaper, thus their use in products has increased dramatically. This trend provides substantial, real time and often continuous flow of information about all aspects of a system. Availability of continuous sensory data improves the ability to diagnose and self-adjust systems for longer and more effective functional life. The same principles apply to patient health monitoring and prognostics.

In addition to proliferation of sensors, substantial amount of data is available from RFID tags. Both active and passive tags are used to track medical equipment, surgical instruments, and patients' movements in medical institutions. These datasets offer tremendous opportunity for clinical analytics and data mining to optimize care team operations, hospital workflows and quality of patient care. In the next sections, an overview of research and literature about medical prediction methods are summarized.

5.8 Prognostics & Prediction in Literature

The American Heritage Dictionary defines *prognostics* as an adjective that relates to prediction or foretelling and as a noun for a sign or symptom indicating the future course of a disease or sign or forecast of some future occurrence. Hippocrates founded the 21 axioms of prognostics some 2400 years ago (MIT 2010). The goal of prognostics is to foretell (predict) the future health (or state) of a system. Health is defined as a state of complete physical, mental, and social well-being.

There are four philosophies pertaining to biological and medical prediction that have evolved through the history of medical prediction. One is grounded in control theory. Decay of human physiology and adverse medical conditions such as Intra-Cranial Pressure (ICP) or carcinogenesis can be viewed as a result of loss of body's control over it critical mechanisms. For example, loss of control over blood flow regulation leads to irregular intracranial pressure; or loss of control over cell cycle that causes altered function of a certain cell population leading to cancer. Medical intervention is viewed as a control action for which the human body is the system. This approach requires a deep understanding of the internal causal models between control mechanisms and human physiology. An example of this approach are the mathematical models using control theory that have employed differential equations to synchronize administration and dosing of chemotherapy drugs with optimum timing of cell life cycle.

The second approach follows the Markov chain model as it considers the disease cycle as a sequence of phases traversed by each physiological subsystem from birth to expiration. For example, a patient with pneumonia starts from healthy, normal state and then follows four stages of Congestion, Red hepatization, Gray hepatization, Resolution (recovery). As another example, a cell cycle consists of growth, DNA synthesis, preparation for division) and division. More recently formulations that model cancer cell growth and decay cycles have been proposed (Hahnfeldt, Danigraphy, Folkman, et al. 1999). These models have considered both deterministic and probabilistic approaches.

The third type of mathematic construct considers the asynchronous nature of biology and uses simulation models. For example, one study applied simulation and statistical process control to estimate occurrence of hospital-acquired infections and to identify medical interventions to prevent transmission of such infections (Limaye, Mastrangelo, Zerr, et al. 2008). Other predictive models in cancer therapy have used stochastic process to predict drug resistance of cancer cells and variability in cell lifetimes. Such a stochastic process is a random walk superimposed on the time-continuous branching process of cell proliferation, namely a branching random walk (Kimmel, Axelrod 2002).

The fourth approach considers the human body as a "gray-box". Since perfect knowledge about each individual's physiology, environmental, genetic and cultural information is not available and in the areas of medicine where our knowledge of clinical evidence is uncertain, one can only rely on predictive models that take data from physiological sensors and laboratory results to make predictions.

Some of the models in this category include the survival analysis provided by Cox Hazard model and Kaplan-Meier estimate. The term survival analysis comes from biomedical research in study of mortality, or patients' survival times from the time of diagnosis of a disease to death. The first survival analysis was developed by John Graunt (Graunt 1662) who for the first time developed life tables based on his birth-death rate observations. Survival analysis is a collection of statistical techniques used to estimate whether an event of interest will occur and at what time. Survival Analysis is known by different names in different disciplines; engineering researchers refer to it as failure-time analysis; sociologists call it event history analysis while economists call it transition analysis.

Among parametric models of survival analysis the Cox hazard function is a popular method. Another method called Kaplan-Meier Estimator is a statistical tool used for non-parametric models where the mathematical equation of the system under study is unknown. Prior to these models, researchers often had to resort to life-table methods.

The Cox hazard model is a partial likelihood method that allows the researcher to estimate the regression coefficients of the proportional hazards model without the need to specify the baseline hazard function. The hazard rate is the probability that if the event in question has not already occurred, it will occur in the next time interval, divided by the length of that interval (Spruance, Reid, Grace, Samore 2004).

Among biomedical researchers the Kaplan Meier Estimator is the tool of choice for survival analysis. Also known as the product-limit estimator, this technique observes all data from all observations by considering survival to any point in time as a series of steps defined by the observed survival and censored times. Some models use Taylor series expansion. It's often used to measure the fraction of patients living for a certain period of time after treatment. One advantage of Kaplan Meier is in its ability to handle censored data, those situations for example where a patient withdraws from a study or the certain start time of the data is not available. Kaplan Meier makes certain assumptions about data independence and uniformity that if violated can result in biased and unreliable data (Tsai, Pollock, Brownie 1999).

Other researchers have adopted a Case Base Reasoning (CBR) method for diagnosis. CBR is an approach for solving a new problem by remembering a previous similar situation and by reusing information and knowledge of that information (Aamodt, Plaza 1994). Since this approach assumes that similar problems have similar solutions, it is considered an appropriate method for practical medical domain that's focused on real cases rather than rules on knowledge to solve problems (Park, Kim, Chun 2008).

The emphasis of this study is on prediction of the individual's short term future health condition and a rule-based prognostics engine that makes such predictions possible. Short term is defined as a time frame that spans from a few seconds to several days from any given moment. The prognostics engine is a computational component that can analyze vast amounts of historical and current physiological data and predict future health of an individual. The predictions are continuous over time based on new, real time data gathered from multiple physiological systems including warnings, alerts, events and precautions.

Admittedly developing mathematical models that make accurate predictions in biology and medicine is challenging but researchers suggest that soon such mathematical models will become a useful adjunct to laboratory experiment (and even clinical trials), and the provision of 'in silico' models will become routine.

Advances in vital-signs monitoring software/hardware, sensor technology, miniaturization, wireless technology and storage allow recording and analysis of large physiological data in a timely fashion (Yu, Liu, McKenna, et al. 2006). This provides both a challenge and an opportunity. The challenge is that the medical decision maker must sift through vast amount of data to make the appropriate care decision. The opportunity is to analyze this large amount of data in real time to provide forecasts about the health of the patient and assist with clinical decisions.

Medical science is grounded in scientific evidence, prior research, experiments and studies that have produced a body of medical knowledge based on generalizations and meta-analysis of research data. Such generalizations explain the causal relationships between risk factors, diseases and diagnosis. There are however gray areas in medical prognostics because many health treatment and screening decisions have no single 'best' choice and because there is scientific uncertainty or the clinical evidence is insufficient (O'Connor, Bennett, Stacey, et al. 2009). In many areas of medical science, the causal relationships are still incompletely understood and controversial. There are environmental, situational, cultural and unique factors that provide specific clinical data about a disease or groups of patients. Although this data is inadequate for making scientific generalizations and clinical evidence, it can provide valuable information to make assessments of individual's health status.

There are situations where collected data is inadequate to make generalizations, the evidence is not full proof or inconclusive, and the collected data requires physician processing and judgment, these fall into a gray area of medical diagnosis and prognosis. This framework presents a model based on multiple algorithms as alternative to linear logistics regression methods to discern patterns and classifications of collected data into specific disease or stages of disease classifications.

A large volume of literature concerning mathematical models to predict biological and medical conditions has been published. But only a few of such works in predictive mathematical tools have found their way into mainstream clinical applications and medical practice. Several reasons are cited for the low adoption of predictive tools: either important biological processes were unrecognized or crucial parameters were not known, or that the mathematical intricacies of predictive models were not understood (Swierniak, Kimmel, Smieja 2009). When such parametric or evidence-based knowledge are not available, predictive model described in this framework can be crucial to make clinical decisions.

The properties of an appropriate mathematical model for medical health condition include: accuracy, prediction, economy, well-posedness and utility (Smye, Clayton 2002). Among constructs used in prior research several distinct mathematical models can be found, such as: Multivariate regression analysis, Markov chains, stochastic processes, Bayesian networks, Fuzzy logic, control theory, discrete event simulation, dynamic programming and Neural Networks.

While control theory has been widely used in systems and other engineering disciplines, it has not widely been applied to prognostics as explained in the next section.

5.9 Control Theoretic Approach to Clinical Prognostics

A system can be broadly defined as an integrated set of elements that accomplish a defined objective (INCOSE 2008). The human body can be considered as a biological system that functions as a collection of interrelated systems. Generally, a control theoretic approach has not been adequately addressed in the literature to the degree that this framework does. In particular the system theory approach in this book covers both feed-forward and feedback mechanisms deliver a richer framework for Prognostics.

Prognostics deals with prediction of some desired quality or characteristic of a system (Kapur 2010). It's based on understanding the science of degradation of the underlying system. The traditional systems control has been predominantly based on feedback: Using the feedback signal, a system's performance could be diagnosed, then adjusted to fix the problem. Obviously, this poses an issue. Correcting the problems after receiving feedback might be too late in certain mission critical systems and in particular when human physiology is considered. Instead, a feed-forward model as exemplified by Prognostics methods would be more desirable. Prognostics methodology is based on two principles: 1) it uses feed-forward models for prediction or forecast of the underlying causes of problems by analyzing feed-forward signals; and 2) it suggests changes in input signal to the system in order to prevent the problem from occurring.

Prognostics and Health Management (PHM) is an engineering discipline that links studies of failure mechanisms to system lifecycle management (Serdar, Goebel, and Lucas, 2008). Other definitions of PHM describe it as a method that permits the assessment of the reliability of a system under its actual application conditions, to determine the advent of failure, and mitigate system risks (Pecht, 2008).

The term "diagnostics" pertains to the detection and isolation of faults or failures. "Prognostics" is the process of predicting a future state (of reliability) based on current and historic conditions (Vichare and Pecht 2006).

Prognostics is the science of predicting the future functionality of a system by estimating the remaining useful life, probability of failure or time to failure for a given system. There are many approaches and modeling frameworks for representing a prognostics system.

Among many methods of prognostics computing the Remaining Useful Life (RUL) of a system is common. RUL can be estimated from historical and operational data collected from a system. Various methods are used to determine system degradation and predict RUL.

Another method is estimating the Probability of Failure (POF). POF is the failure probability distribution of the system or a component. Additionally, it's common to study Time to failure (TTF), the time a component is expected to fail. TTF defines the time when a system no longer meets its design specifications.

Prognostics and Reliability are interrelated. Reliability is defined as the probability that product will perform its intended function, satisfactorily for its intended life when operating under specified condition (Kapur 2010). A clinical definition can be derived from this technical description; Reliability is the probability that a patient will not develop certain medical complication during the length stay under medical care of the care provider(s). Reliability is measured by several indicators such as Mean Time Between Failure (MTBF), Failure rate and Percentiles of Life. Each measurement can be computed from corresponding equations that are derived from empirical and statistical distribution functions. Additional treatment of Reliability can be found from text by Kapur and Lamberson (Kapur, Lamberson 1977).

Prognostics models can be classified into three general types (Eklund 2009; Hines 2009; Peysson et al. 2009). Type I is reliability based. It applies the traditional time to failure analysis by tracking a population of failures and using statistical methods for the estimation of reliability. Some typical life distributions that are used in this type of prognostics include Weibull, exponential and normal distributions. Type I prognostic methods does not incorporate the real time monitoring of operating conditions or environmental conditions.

Type II methods, also known as the stressor-based approaches consider the operational and environmental condition data. Type II considers the failures of a system in its operating environment to provide an average remaining life of a component. Some of the environmental data might include temperature, vibration, humidity and load. The proportional hazard model is an example of a type II prognostic model. Knowing the causes, one can predict reliability of a system. The simplest model in this approach is the regression model: given the operating and environmental conditions, one can predict the system failure and remaining useful life by a regression equation.

Type III prognostic methods are condition-based, namely they characterize the lifetime of a system in operation within its specific environment. They estimate the remaining life of a specific component or the entire system. Among methods used in Type III prognostics are the General Path Model (GPM), Neural Network models, Expert systems, Fuzzy rule-based systems, and multi-state analysis. Another example of type III approach is the cumulative Damage model.

The cumulative damage model tracks the irreversible accumulation of damage in systems or components. The statistical cumulative damage model considers the number of possible damage states and a transition matrix (for representing a multi-state Markov Chain) to provide a damage prediction for multiple cyclical loads.

It's the Type III Prognostics method using Artificial Neural Network and other algorithms that this framework employs to continuously predict a patient's health status at regular time intervals.

Chapter 6

Analytics Methods in Predictive Medicine

Neural Networks have been used successfully to predict future onset of diseases such as recurrence of various types of cancer, cardiology illnesses and to assist physicians with prognostic and decision support. These studies have offered long term predictions for patient health conditions, typically forecasting the disease-free or disease recurrence in the future ranging from a few months to several years.

Artificial Neural networks (ANNs) are parallel computational methods by interconnecting artificial neurons. They're ideal for solving non-linear problems that come with a long list and diverse types of input variables. ANNs are adaptive to specific problems and can be trained for pattern matching or classification. An ANN model can be trained by mapping a disease to a known set of input clinical measurements and then later be applied to a new patient. The trained model can match the input measurements of the patient to presence or absence of a disease. The model can even classify the patient's clinical measurements into various stages of a disease.

Since early 1980's, Artificial Neural networks have been applied successfully to several prediction problems in business, engineering and medicine (Delen 2009). One of the most popular models is the Multi-Layer Perceptron (MLP) with back propagation, essentially a supervised learning algorithm. It's been shown that ANN models using MLP algorithm are capable of learning arbitrarily complex non-linear functions to arbitrary accurate levels (Hornik 1990). The MLP is essentially a collection of non-linear neurons connected together by weighted links in a feed-forward multi-layer structure. Among highly accurate models, Support Vector Machines (SVMs) have been proposed (Delen 2009). SVM algorithm is not regarded as an artificial neural network model, but it's been included in the ensemble for its solver capability. Most recent algorithms use Levenberg-marquardt methods proposed by Levenberg and Marquardt that are highly accurate as well as computationally fast ANN models (Wilamowski & Chen, 1999). Support Vector Machines are not regarded as Neural Networks, but they can be used as solver method in a Neural Network model.

Medical research has shown that certain life-threatening conditions exhibit early indicators in physiological data. A study conducted on improving neonatal intensive care units (NICU) (Blount 2010) provided interpretations of multiple streams of clinical and physiological data to detect medically significant conditions that precede the onset of medical complications for neonatal patients.

In another study (Webber 1994), A neural network model was trained on EEG data. The input consisted of 49 channels of real time EEG data to detect epilepsy spikes. The study showed that ANNs offer a practical solution for automated detection of real time epileptiform discharges using inexpensive computers.

ANNs have been shown to be a valuable tool to the clinical diagnosis of myocardial infarction (Baxt 1994). The model used in one study was trained on 351 patients admitted for high likelihood of having myocardial infarction. It was prospectively tested on 331 consecutive patients presenting to the ED department with anterior chest pain. The network was able to distinguish patients with from those without acute myocardial infarction at a slightly higher sensitivity than physicians' diagnosis for those patients.

In another study of patients in Intensive Care Units (ICUs), an ANN model was shown to be more effective than logistic regression model for predicting outcome of care (Dybowski, et al. 1996). The ANN model was applied in the clinical setting of systemic inflammatory response syndrome and hemodynamic shock on 258 patients. The outcome evaluated was death during that hospital admission. The best performing ANN model was trained after 7 training iterations.

In cancer treatment cases, ANNs have become a popular tool for predicting outcomes (Dayhoff, DeLeo 2001). At one institution (Bottaci, et al. 1997) six different ANN models were developed to predict outcome of individual patients who were diagnosed with colorectal cancer to predict death within 9, 12, 15, 18, 21, and 24 months. Results showed that ANNs were able to detect outcome more accurately than the then available clinicopathological methods.

Other research conducted in the breast cancer patients (Ravdin, Clark 2005) suggest that ANNs can be trained to recognize patients with high and low risk of recurrent disease and death. Moreover, their study showed that by coding time as one of the prognostic variables, an ANN can be used to predict patient outcome over time. In particular ANN models can make a series of predictions about probability of relapse at different times of follow up, allowing clinicians to draw survival probability curves for individual patients.

In another study a set of patients' mammography tests were interpreted by radiologists and by an ANN model (Floyd, et al. 1994). The model was more accurate in detecting breast cancer patients than radiologists. A more comprehensive overview of application of neural networks in decision support of cancer found 396 studies and found that overall ANNs add more benefit to making decisions in the field of cancer (Lisboa et al. 2005).

Several studies have compared the accuracy of ANNs with Logistic regression models, but after a meta-analysis the conclusions are mixed. Some papers (Delen 2009) show that ANNs are far more accurate, but a few papers find both methods comparable for medical prediction (Adams, Wert 2005). The next section reviews the validation and viability measurements that are used as criteria to select the most appropriate model.

6.1 Model Viability and Validation Methods

Model validation and verification are important steps for providing confidence and credibility in the model's results. Verification (ensures that the model performs as intended) and validation (ensures that the model represents and correctly reproduces the behaviors of the real world system) are essential elements of model development for practical applications (Macal 2005). Model verification deals with building the model right. Validations deals with building the right model.

The goal of validation is to ensure that the model addressed the right problem, provided accurate information about the system being modeled. One of the dangers to modeling validity is "overfitting" the model to a given data set, where the model is fitted to a specific dataset. Overfitting can occur when important elements of the model reflect randomness in the data rather than underlying model drivers. To overcome this limitation, researchers have employed techniques such as cross-validation, or keeping a "hold-out" random data sample to perform testing on a separate data set. In addition, researchers have considered accuracy measures of the model using prior data as the expected results.

Three aspects of validity are advised:

1. Calibration - agreement between observed probabilities and predicted probabilities,
2. Discrimination - ability of the model to distinguish between different outcomes,

3. Clinical usefulness - ability of the model to improve decision making process.

There are two types of validation, the internal validation and external validation. Internal validation uses techniques such as cross validation and boot-strapping to assess the performance in samples of the same population. External validation is the process of measuring performance of prediction model in samples from different populations such as patients from other locations. With cross-validation technique, the model is developed in a randomly selected part of the data sample and test on the rest of the sample, then the process is repeated several times and the average is computed as the estimate of performance. With boot-strapping technique, a sample of the same size as the development sample is randomly selected with replacement, the model then is developed in the boot-strap samples and testing on those not included in the boot-strap samples.

Tests that measure clinical usefulness include accuracy, sensitivity, specificity and decrease in weighed false classifications. Tests that measure discrimination include Receiver Operating Characteristic (ROC) curve, a plot of model *sensitivity* vs. *(1 – specificity)*. Finally tests that measure calibration include calibration plot and average absolute different between observed frequencies and predicted probabilities. These measurements are defined and employed in this framework as described in the upcoming chapters.

External validation requires clinical trials and specific clinical design of experiments that are outside the scope of this framework. However, internal validity test is covered in this book on all four analytical models and the five derived ensemble that are developed for the predictive framework.

6.2 History of Analytical Methods in Medical Prognostics

A vast majority of mathematical models in medicine are used in diagnosis. Models to make prediction using prognostics have not been fully explored. Among those that did address predictive analytics, many required and made assumptions about the type of data and distribution. For example, many studies assumed normality in their data set. Most have relied on a single model to make predictions. Little attention has been paid to developing a framework for prediction of patient health status using prognostic methods on these large data sets. This framework develops and explores a multi-model prognostics framework for prediction and demonstrates its feasibility as a systemic prognostics method to predict patient health status.

Traditionally, the two most commonly used data mining techniques are Linear Discriminant Analysis (LDA) and logistic regression to construct classification models. However, one criticism leveled against LDA has been due to assumption about the categorical nature of the data and the fact that the covariance matrices of different classes are unlikely to be equal. Research in cancer data analysis has demonstrated that generally ANNs are more accurate than linear logistic regression models in predicting cases of new or recurrent cancer (Delen 2009).

From a survey of literature from 1970s to present, it's established that more attention has been given to decision support and diagnoses and less to predicting short term medical health condition of individual patients. The most successful predictive methods in literature are model-free approaches using neural networks and fuzzy sets (Kodell, Pearce, Baek, et al. 2009, and Arthi, Tamilarasi 2008).

CPRs are typically arrived at through logistic regression type of analysis. Logistic regression is a special form of linear regression models that allows non-numeric input variables (namely allows categorical data). It's used for classification or prediction with the probability that an event will occur by fitting data to a logit function (or a natural log function) logistic curve.

Logistic Regression (LR) is a generalization of linear regression. It's used as the means to predict binary or multi-class dependent variables. Since the response variable is discrete, it cannot be modeled directly by linear regression. Instead, logistic regression rather than predicting a point estimate of the event itself, builds the model to predict the odds of its occurrence. When predicting the occurrence or no-occurrence of a disease, basically a two-class problem, if the odds are greater than 50%, it implies that the case is assigned to the class designated as 1, otherwise as 0. The LR assumes that the response variable (the log of odds) is linear in the coefficients of the predictor variables. In addition, the LR models do not select the best inputs and the modeler must select the right inputs and specify their relationship to the response variable (Delen 2009). These are among limitations to prior research that have employed Logistic Regression.

Classification trees (also referred to as decision trees) are used to predict membership of cases in the classes of categorical dependent variable based on their measurements on predictor variables. Researchers prefer classification trees over the traditional statistical tools when assumptions about data distribution cannot be met or the researcher seeks exploratory study of data classification. Classification trees have been used in medical studies (Breiman, Friedman, Olshen, Stone 1984) to aid in diagnosis. They form hierarchical models of data with branches in a tree-like structure that lead to specific diagnosis. The pitfalls with these methods are shown to be related to their linear approach and errors associated with initial choice of data that forms the tree classification.

Historically, most predictive methods have relied on either a single model for prediction and/or on linear methods for prediction and generalizing CPR rules. While predictive models using ANN have been reported in the literature, such models provide long term predictions that span over several years in the future, and do not focus on short term predictions.

Prior research has predominantly limited their model validation to a few criteria, such as sensitivity, specificity and ROC calculations. They have limited their models to only one ANN model or to the algorithm that produced the best results. They have not compared results of four ANN models along these and other validation measurements which this framework has addressed.

Given these limitations, this framework proposes a multi-model prognostics framework along with an oracle to select the most appropriate model for a given disease prediction. Furthermore, this framework compares a wide range of validity measures on all four models and ensemble of these models. The use of multi-model prediction and in particular using ensemble of models combined with an oracle overseer as explored in this framework are novel approaches in clinical data analytics.

6.3 Statistical Analysis of DRG Classification

Statistical methods used for basic clinical analytics include algorithms that identify trends, measure expected value, and identify outliers and variability. The NHS Casemix Design Authority has published several guidelines for statistical analysis of clinical data and DRG classifications which are referenced here (NHS Casemix 2009). These statistical tools are briefly addressed here for DRG classification, but apply to a host of other variables in healthcare.

Identification of outlier LoS variability

Clinical Intelligence reports can include summary statistics (mean, median and percentiles) for each DRG by provider and Length of Stay (LoS) distribution for each DRG can be produced in order to identify DRGs with unusual LoS distributions, for example bimodal or irregular distributions, or those with a higher than expected proportion of outliers.

Often a regression line provides the basis for determining the best line that fits a number of data points in a scatter diagram. Given the regression line, one of the techniques to identify outliers is to define an acceptable range above and below the regression line, forming an acceptable band. These upper and lower lines define trim-points. All data points that fall outside of this band (outside of trim-points) are regarded outliers.

Measurement of intra-DRG cost variability

DRG values can be analyzed using appropriate statistical methods compared to nationally collected cost data in order to determine the degree of cost variation both between and within DRGs

Determining DRGs with disproportionate numbers of outliers

An outlier is defined as an observation that is numerically distant from the rest of the data. In DRG terms it is a patient episode of care with LoS greater than the trim-point. The proportion of episodes that are outliers for either LoS or cost can be determined for each DRG after calculating the DRGs upper trim-point.

Reduction in Variance (RIV) - Inter Group Variation

RIV statistic is used to measure the explanatory power of casemix systems, i.e. the proportion of total LoS variation explained by the groups. A value of 0% means that the classification explains none of the variance in the dependent variable (e.g. LoS or cost), whilst 100% means it explains all of the variance. 100%, whilst theoretically possible, would suggest that all the data in each group have the same LoS/cost. Typical results for LoS would be 30-40% whilst cost would be 60-70%.

The RIV, often expressed as R^2 to describe the predictive validity of the classifications, is calculated to describe the explanatory power of the grouping classifications. The unadjusted form of the calculation of RIV is the inverse of the ratio of the whole sum of squares (WSS) and the total sum of squares (TSS), expressed as a percentage.

$$R^2 = 1 - \frac{WSS}{TSS}$$

Where WSS = whole sum of squares

             TSS = total sum of squares

$$WSS = \sum_{j=1}^{k}\sum_{i=1}^{n_j}(x_{ij} - \bar{x}_j)^2 \qquad TSS = \sum_{j=1}^{k}\sum_{i=1}^{n_j}(x_{ij} - \bar{x})^2$$

Where k = the number of groups

             n_j = the number of cases in group j

             x_{ij} = value of case i in group j

             $\bar{x}_j$ = mean of group j

             $\bar{x}$ = overall mean

Coefficient of Variation (CV) – Intra group variation

Whie the RIV statistic gives a result to be applied across groups, a statistic is required to measure the within-group variability or homogeneity. The ratio of standard deviation (SD) to the arithmetic mean of a group, or CV gives a measure of the relative variability within a single group.

$$CV = \frac{SD}{\bar{x}} = \frac{\sqrt{\sum_{i=1}^{n}(x_i - \bar{x})^2 / n}}{\bar{x}}$$

Where   SD = standard deviation of the group

$\bar{x}$ = mean of group

x_i = value of case i in the group

n = the number of cases in the group

The CV is reported for a group to describe its homogeneity. A value of 0 would indicate that a group has no variance from the mean (i.e. standard deviation is equal to 0), while a CV value for a group above 1.00 would indicate heterogeneity within the group, where the standard deviation is greater than the mean. We would anticipate that the more homogenous a DRG is, the more likely it is that the underlying DRG Design is robust. Caution should be used when the mean is close to zero as CV may be sensitive to small changes in the mean.

Classification and Regression Tree:

Classification and regression tree (CART) is a set of techniques for classification and prediction. The purpose of the analyses via tree-building algorithms is to determine a set of *if-then* logical (split) conditions that permit accurate classification of cases. When applied to DRG classification, given a resource variable e.g. LoS or Cost, the algorithm will identify groupings that best differentiate between high and low resource cases, using any variable in the dataset. For instance, within a given dataset, it may find firstly that there are some diagnosis codes that have high resource and some that have low resource. Within each diagnostic group it may then find that age further differentiates, and add further splits on the basis of age.

Chapter 7

Clinical Intelligence Prediction Framework

The clinical intelligence model presented in this framework provides a feed-forward model to make predictions based on models trained on prior patient data. A prediction is a form of speculation about a state in the future. A prediction is foretelling a medical event or disease when the ingredients for that medical event are in place but have not combined to affect their significance in form of a disease yet. A marker is the recognition that the ingredients for a medical event are in place and have indeed combined to result in form of a disease but in lower and milder yet measurable doses.

Since clinical data changes from population to population, by geography and temporal time stamps, using a single model is often inadequate to achieve a high level of accuracy and resiliency to changes in data. Hence, I've proposed using an ensemble of models and an overseer program (which I call an Oracle) to provide a composite set of results from multiple models. Given different data sets with different data sizes and data characteristic, each model can perform better (more accuracy and specificity as will be explained later). This framework is the ensemble (also known as the committee of models) program. Figure 7.1 illustrates this framework.

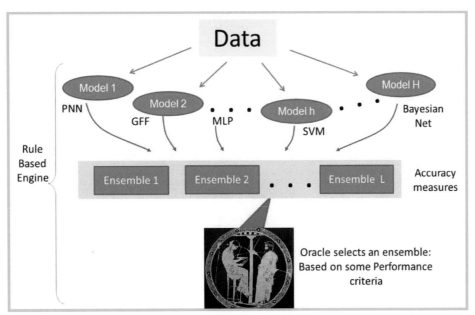

Fig. 7.1 – The Ensemble (Committee of Model) Framework for a Robust Clinical Intelligence System

The precursor to a disease is known as risk factors in medicine. Thus, the spectrum of medical predictions starts with risk factors, leading to prediction, and then on to markers and finally to the occurrence of the disease or medical event itself. The following graph illustrates the chronology of events and progression of the individual's health status from risk factors towards confirmed stage of disease or medical event manifestation. The distance between time ticks are arbitrary and vary among individuals. The medical prediction models must take into account the prior history, risk factors, markers and the medical intervention as inputs to the model. Once medical intervention is applied, patients' physiological data is expected to reflect recovery and return of patient health condition into the desired range. Such recovery can be expected and compared against measured changes in the patients' health status. The intent of this framework is to study the viability of using ANN to make predictions in the time scale shown in Figure 2.

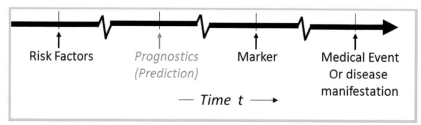

Figure 7.2 - Progression of individual health condition

7.1 An Overview of Predictive Analytical Models

There are five evolving philosophies pertaining to biological and medical prediction: One is grounded in control theory. Decay of human physiology and adverse medical conditions such as Intra-Cranial Pressure (ICP) or carcinogenesis can be viewed as a result of loss of body's control over it critical mechanisms. For example, loss of control over blood flow regulation leads to irregular intracranial pressure; or loss of control over cell cycle that causes altered function of a certain cell population leading to cancer. Medical intervention is viewed as a control action on the specific physiological subsystem, for which the human body is the general system. This approach requires a deep understanding of the internal causal models between control mechanisms and human physiology. The mathematical models using control theory have employed differential equations to synchronize administration and dosing of chemotherapy drugs with optimum timing of cell life cycle. Such models have offered treatment protocols that maximize the effect of drug dosages on cell subpopulation while minimizing impact on healthy cells.

The second approach follows the Markov chain model as it considers the disease cycle as a sequence of phases traversed by each physiological subsystem from birth to expiration. For example, a patient with pneumonia starts from healthy, normal state and then follows four stages of Congestion, Red hepatization, Gray hepatization, Resolution (recovery). As another example, a cell cycle consists of G1 (or growth), S (for DNA Synthesis), G2(preparation for division) and M(division). A similar model in this category is the Gompetz Curve, a sigmoidal function which has been used to predict cancer cell growth. More recently formulations that model cancer cell growth and decay cycles have been proposed (Hahnfeldt, Danigraphy, Folkman, et al. 1999). These models have considered both deterministic and probabilistic approaches.

The third type of mathematic construct considers the asynchronous nature of biology and thus this approach uses simulation models. For example, one study applied simulation and statistical process control to estimate occurrence of hospital-acquired infections and to identify medical interventions to prevent transmission of such infections (Limaye, Mastrangelo, Zerr, et al. 2008).

The fourth approach such as those used as predictive models in cancer therapy have used stochastic process to predict drug resistance of cancer cells and variability in cell lifetimes. Such a stochastic process is a random walk superimposed on the time-continuous branching process of cell proliferation, namely a branching random walk (Kimmel, Axelrod 2002).

144

The fifth approach considers the human body as a black box. Since perfect knowledge about each individual's physiology, environmental, genetic and cultural information are not known and in the areas of medicine where our knowledge of clinical evidence is uncertain, one must rely on predictive models that take physiological sensor data and laboratory results to make predictions.

7.2 Conceptual Model

This framework offers a feed-forward model based on Prognostics and Health Management methodology. The model consists of several key components: Input, output, measured data, database of prior cases, a prognostics engine and the feed-forward signal as shown in Figure 3. The rule-based engine, essentially a classification tool uses ANN models to make prediction.

The model proposed by this framework considers the medical treatment plan as an input to the patients' physiological system. Represented by *u(t)*, medical treatment plan involves some set of medications, procedures and care protocols prescribed by the physician. The patients' physiology is the process that produces a clinical outcome at time *t*, shown by *y(t)*. The patients' clinical outcome is the output or the response variable. The outcome is a vector of single or multiple states of health for that patient. The model is shown in Figure 7.3.

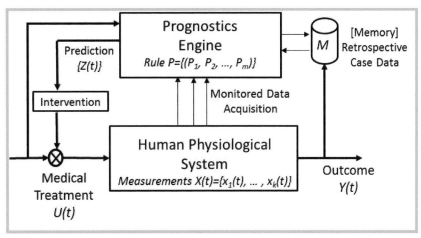

Figure7. 1 - The Medical Prognostics Model

The input variable can be shown as:

$$U(t) = \{u_1(t), \ u_2(t), \dots, u_q(t)\} \tag{1}$$

The output, known as the clinical outcome represents the patient's health status. This is represented by the response variable and defined as:

$$Y(t) = \{y_1(t), \ y_2(t), \dots, y_m(t)\} \tag{2}$$

The input vector *U(t)* indicates which of medical protocols, procedures and treatments are applied at time *t*. Each *u_i(t)* indicates a unique treatment defined by CPT codes for time *t*. The complete list of procedures is codified and can be found in a library of Current Procedural Terminology (CPT) code which includes approximately 8,700 unique procedures (American Medical Association 2010).

145

Vector *Y(t)* is the response variable, representing a set of diseases at time *t*. The diseases correspond to ICD-9 diagnosis codes found in ICD-9 library (WHO 2012). A response variable $Y_i(t)$ indicates the value or stage of disease *i* at time *t*. The value can be binary (1 or 0, namely True or False, indicating the presence or absence of a disease), or a discreet value (indicating the stage or class of a disease). For example, let's select a variable from the set *Y(t)*, say variable $y_{18}(t)$, to denote the presence of lupus. Lupus has five stages. When the value of $Y_{18}(t)$ is 3, it indicates that lupus is present and it's in stage 3. But if the value of $Y_{18}(t)$ is 0, it implies the presence of lupus for the patient is negative.

The internal physiological system measurements consisting of clinical and vital sign data can cover a wide range of measurements including lab results, Radiology exams and real time information. These measurements are represented by the set *X(t)*:

$$X(t) = \{x_1(t), x_2(t), \dots, x_k(t)\} \tag{3}$$

The medical prognostics model employs a prognostics engine that consists of a set of pre-trained mathematical models to predict specific outcome for time *(t + t₁)*. Each mathematical model represents a dedicated rule for predicting a specific disease value. The rules are defined by the set *P*. In other words, *P* is the set of prediction rules, namely the set of trained ANN models that make the disease predictions. The prognostics engine works as follows: it collects vital clinical data from the patients' physiological system and makes a prediction for *t₁* minutes in advance, for time *(t + t₁)*. The prognostics engine delivers a prediction vector *{Z}* that can be used to modify the medical treatment plan *u(t)*.

Let's define clinical outcome *Y(t)* as a function of medical intervention, physiological measurements and unknown cause-and-effect variables that can be accumulated into error $\hat{e}$:

$$Y(t) = F(\{X(t)\}, \{U(t)\}, \{Z(t)\}, \hat{e}) \tag{4}$$

The prediction rules are trained based on prior evidence and formed from retrospective collection of past patient data. The set of prognostic rules can be defined by:

$$P = \{p_1, p_2, \dots, p_m\} \tag{5}$$

The prediction rules are models defined by analyzing retrospective cases. Each prediction rule is defined by a model that transforms the input data set *X(t)* to a particular disease Y_i. The prognostics engine works continuously by monitoring real time patient data and simultaneously applying multiple mathematical algorithms p_i every so many established minutes such that it can make predictions about occurrence of diseases or adverse events occurring in the near future. The prognostics vector *Z(t)* consists of *m* values, indicating predictions about disease type and value for that disease shown by $z_i(t)$:

$$Z(t) = \{z_1(t), \dots, z_m(t)\} \tag{6}$$

The medical intervention, retrospective case information and monitored data can be mathematically described as sets of variables. One can express prediction as a function of multiple variables including the input clinical data and medical intervention. Prediction is a mapping between new input data and an outcome from a set of retrospective cases. The most suitable mapping is selected by a classification function defined by the set of rules p_i for disease *i*. The classification function maps a set of input variable data pattern with a specific disease using rules p_i. Each rule p_i is trained to detect disease i, so there is a one-to-one association between each rule p_i and disease i. Prediction for time $(t+t_1)$ is a vector of predicted disease values:

$$z_i(t + t_1) = p_i\{X(1), \dots, X(t), U(1), \dots, U(t), Y(1), \dots, Y(t)\} \tag{7}$$

where physiological data set collected from the patient is represented by vector $X(t)$; medical treatment plans are selected from a set of treatment plans shown as $U(t)$; and retrospective cases are represented by M as the set of prior relationships established between physiological data and outcome. The relationship between prediction and predicted disease at time $t+t_1$ can be shown as:

$$Prediction_{(t)} = Z(t), \xrightarrow{yields} \{Y_1(t + t_1), \dots, Y_i(t + t_1), \dots, Y_m(t + t_1)\} \tag{8}$$

The goal of This framework is to identify the appropriate mathematical model $P(X, U, Y)$ that selects the appropriate prediction from a set of possible outcomes, in other words determine the value of $Y_i(t+t_1)$ as True, False or other discreet values indicating the stage of disease. The value of $Y_i(t+t_1)$ determines the classification for a given patient and answers the question of which disease classification the patient belongs to. Each p_i model is a mapping function developed based on historical data patterns that maps the input data to a specific outcome. The function $P(X, U, Y)$ is a classification function that selects one or more clinical disease states from the set Y.

The model is intended to be used by physicians. A typical use-case scenario is as follows: A physician, the user of this tool, will train the ANN model based on a-priori data and outcomes. When the ANN model is trained, the physician can apply the model to new patient data. When the ANN model is applied once, it provides diagnostic and prognostic classifications. The ANN model can be trained over a time interval taking into account a time series of clinical data points. The model can be set up to run repetitively every few minutes for one or more patients to provide real-time and ongoing predictions about upcoming presence or absence of a clinical condition. The next section describes the four ANN models and their characteristics that are employed in this framework.

7.3 Artificial Neural Network models

The power of artificial networks comes in its ability to detect patterns, including those complicated situations when the traditional statistical analysis would take an inordinate amount of time that would render them impractical (Monterola, Lim, et al 2002).

An artificial neural network is a network of interconnected processing elements that can classify patterns from a set of input data. Unlike the traditional computer architectures, known as von-Neumann computers, ANNs are trained, rather than programmed. When a set of data is fed into an ANN model if there is a pattern in the data, the ANN 'learns' them. Once the pattern is learned, the ANN model can classify a new set of data into the appropriate categories.

The suitable predictive mathematical model must offer accuracy and simplicity to learn from prior cases and easily be extensible to apply new data to make predictions about a patient's health condition. The four ANN algorithms selected in this framework are established through literature among the most commonly used and accurate neural network models for prediction and classification. Each model has certain relative strength and weakness depending on the input data and computational constraints (Principe 2011). This framework developed four models for comparison. The models are:

1) PNN - Probabilistic Neural Networks are four layer networks. They classify data in a non-parametric method and are less sensitive to outlier data. These models are known for performing well when datasets are small.

2) SVM – Support Vector Machine networks. SVM performs classification by constructing a two-layer network that defines a hyperplane that separates data into multiple classifications. This method is generally regarded among more accurate classification models. Support Vector Machines are not regarded as Neural Networks, but they can be used as solver method in a Neural Network model.

3) MLP trained with LM – Multi-layer perceptron with Levenberg-Marquardt algorithm, a gradient descent approach with variable step modification. This algorithm is regarded as computationally efficient method.

4) GFN (Generalized Feed-forward network) trained with LM – Generalized multi-layer feed-forward network with Levenberg-Marquardt algorithm. These models typically perform well when datasets are large and many data cases are available.

In order to make predictions on time-series data, a time-lag recurring network variation may be used for each of the above algorithms. The time-lag recurring network is essentially a time-series modeling approach that shifts the prediction several iterations forward in time and provides results of several samples ahead.

Different neural network models use different learning rules, but in general they all determine pattern statistics from a set of training examples and then classify new data according to the trained rules. Stated differently, a trained neural network model classifies (or maps) a set of input data to a specific disease from a set of diseases.

7.4 Analytic Model Comparison and Evaluation

Feasibility and utility of the model is gauged against five criteria of accuracy, well-posedness, utility, adaptability and economy. Each criterion is explored further in the following sections.

Accuracy

Accuracy of a model is the degree of closeness of the model's results to the system's actual value. Precision of a model is the degree to which repeated runs of the model under unchanged conditions produces the same results. Since the model is trained on retrospective data, it's easy to evaluate the prediction accuracy of the model to the actual clinical outcomes from prior retrospective patient cases. Analysis about accuracy will include measurements such as calibration (agreement between predicted probability and observed outcome frequencies), discrimination (ability to distinguish between patients with and without the disease), sensitivity (proportion of patients who are correctly diagnosed as having the disease), specificity (proportion of healthy patients who are correctly diagnosed with negative result), likelihood ratio (LR, how much the odds of disease change based on a positive or negative test result) and receiver operating characteristic (ROC, a plot of sensitivity vs. one minus specificity) curves.

This study evaluates model validity and accuracy through internal validation using clinical outcomes of prior patient data obtained from retrospective studies. Clinical validation and impact analysis on prospective cases are outside the scope of this framework. This book proposes an oracle schema to select the most accurate model, or to select an ensemble of models that provide higher accuracy of prediction.

Comparing prediction accuracy of ANN and other statistical models requires standards for comparison using classification performance indices. These indices include Receiver Operating Characteristic (ROC, a plot of sensitivity vs. one minus specificity) curve, Area Under Receiver-Operating Characteristics (AUROC, an overall measure of accuracy that measures the area under ROC curve and where bigger area indicates higher accuracy), sensitivity, specificity, accuracy and positive predictive value (PPV, probability that someone with a positive test result to actually have the disease) and negative predictive value (NPV, probability that someone with a negative test result to actually not have the disease) (Bourdes, et al. 2011).

Sensitivity measures the fraction of positive cases classified as positive. Specificity measures the fraction of negative cases classified as negative.

AUROC is a good overall measure of predictive accuracy of a model. It represents the area under the ROC curve, a measure of how well a model can distinguish between disease and normal groups. An AUROC value near 0.50 suggests no discrimination, namely one can flip a coin to decide. But, an AUROC close to 1.0 is considered excellent discrimination (Linder, Geier, Kolliker 2004). The single measure for accuracy comparison of models and committee of models will be AUC, Area Under Characteristic curve.

Well-posedness: Stability & Immunity to small perturbations of input data

Generally a mathematical model is regarded well-posed if it meets Hadamard's three criteria: 1) the model has a solution, 2) the solution in unique, and 3) the solution depends continuously on the data (Lucchetti 2006). Conversely an ill posed mathematical model has initial, or boundary data, where an infinitesimal perturbation can grow unbounded away from the unperturbed solution. Generally, if it can be proven that the solution is uniformly bounded everywhere then it is well posed. But on the other hand it's possible to have unbounded solutions which are not ill posed. Since most classification problems include local optima as possible solutions, they're not regarded as well-posed. However to overcome this limitation, I've applied genetic algorithm version of ANN such that the solutions consider multiple optima and avoid the local optima trap. Therefore some level of regularization is necessary for the other models. In other words, one must know how to use additional assumptions to create a well-posed behavior in these Artificial Neural networks.

Utility: Practicality in the medical workflow

Once the model is trained, the model can be set up to run automatically at certain time intervals ranging from every minute to every several hours. It's practical to have all four models trained in advance and run them in parallel. An Oracle program can provide the most accurate prediction by polling the four ANN model results. The results can be filtered by the Oracle such that if the occurrence of a disease is detected, the Oracle program would send an alert to the physician.

Adaptability: Ability to handle new evidence, i.e. new data values and data types

ANNs are able to adapt to new data sets, additional variables and all data types. It's recommended that an ANN model be retrained after every few months to adapt to new data and overcome the temporal, environmental and demographic changes that might occur in patients. In this framework, the Memory module collects and maintains clinical data. ANN models can be re-trained as new data become available from the Memory module.

Economy: Cost of computation and timeliness of prediction

In computing, the computational cost of algorithms is determined by an asymptotic number of computations required for an algorithm to complete. The complexity measure of neural network algorithms provides an upper limit on the worst case scenario when the input variables and number of cases grow large. The computational cost of an algorithm is a function of number of steps to compute (time complexity), memory size (space complexity) and length of algorithm. In ANNs, the number of computations is a time complexity, the number of perceptrons is a measure of space complexity and the number of weights is a measure of algorithm length. The complexity of ANNs has been shown to be NP-complete, namely given enough information and hardware, they can predict any input-output function in a finite time (Kon, Plaskota 2000).

The four classification and prediction models used in the case study were trained in under 5 minutes of CPU time and under one hour elapsed time on an average personal computer. The cost of computation is not extreme for a new prediction and can be completed within less than 2 minutes for cases of comparable dataset sizes, such as the case studied in this framework. This is to show that many of the algorithms can be trained quickly and many clinical intelligence analytics studies are within the realm of computational power available.

The development of the four models and their mathematical equations is covered in the next chapter.

Chapter 8

PROGNOSTICS MODEL AND FRAMEWORK DEFINTION

Prognostics is the science of predicting the future functionality of a system by estimating the remaining useful life, probability of failure or time to failure for a given system. The root of the word "system" comes from the Latin word "systema" and the Greek word "systema", meaning a whole compounded of several parts (Merriam-Webster 2011). The closest engineering definition for a system is given as "a group of interacting, interrelated, or interdependent elements forming a complex whole" (Dictionary.com 2012). According to Zadeh and Desoer, to study a system, one defines a simpler representation in form of a model (or models) that represent the physical system (Zadeh and Desoer 1963). Given a model, a mathematical representation and notation for the system can be developed. Finally one can analyze the model by considering its properties, capabilities and its limitations; these three goals are regarded as the task of system theory (Zadeh, Desoer 1963).

Control theory involves the study of "control" or "regulation" of an object or process. Control systems can be classified into either "open" or "closed" systems. In the "open-loop" system the goal is to program the system in advance to give a desired output. This is the notion of a feed-forward mechanism. The closed-loop system relies on feedback from the system's output in order to make adjustment to the input so the system gives the desired output (Wishart 1969).

A control system consists of certain variables that affect the system, the output of the system called output, a controller that compares the input with the output and uses the difference to activate the control elements. The signal that returns the output to the controller is called feedback.

In an open loop system, the goal of properly regulating the system can be attempted by using a feed-forward signal. Since it's possible to monitor and measurement certain variables of the system, one can use those measurements to make adjustments the input (instead of adjusting the control elements) to ensure the system gives the desired output.

In control theory, an interesting question is the level of stability that can be achieved, and optimal control. In this framework a hybrid control system is proposed, consisting of both feed-forward and feedback control. Our goal is to apply control theoretic approach to prognostics. Prognostics is the science of predicting the future functionality of a system by estimating the remaining useful life, probability of failure or time to failure for a given system or component in the system.

8.2 Control Model

In this paper, notations consistent with control system research are used (Kapur 2010). A typical system consists of input r and response variable (or output) represented by y. If the researcher has perfect knowledge about this system, and knows the transfer function $f_o(r) = y$, then inputs r can be determined as $r = f_o^{-1}(y)$. Assuming the system (transfer function) is known; one can predict the response variable y and adjust the inputs r to maintain the output within the desired range. This is the ideal process as shown in Figure 8.1.

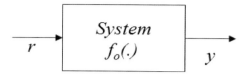

Figure 8.1: The ideal "Perfect" Process

A perfect prognostics is the situation where the researcher knows the transfer function and a perfect knowledge of the system is available. Since the desired output **y** is known, one can determine how input **r** should be adjusted. However, there are challenges to achieving this goal:

1. The inverse problem is not unique and not easy to determine.
2. There is often lack knowledge (or there is uncertainty) about our model.
3. The real world systems might be very complex and cause output **y** to appear as random variable.

In real world, not all systems offer a perfectly known transfer function. Since the causes of variation can't be perfectly known, one must attribute the variation in **y** to disturbance represented by **d**, as shown in Figure 8.2.

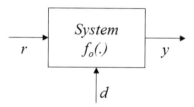

Figure 8.2 - Process with disturbance **d** causing variability in output **y**

One way to correct for the effects of disturbance and variation is to use feedback as shown in Figure 8.3. Feedback signal is represented by signal **v**. In a basic feedback loop, the output is returned back to a controller to adjust the input. But using feedback to adjust input proves to be too late for adjusting the input in a timely manner.

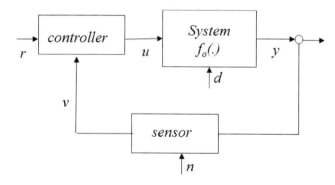

Fig. 8.3: Process with feedback loop to reduce variability in output y

The traditional approaches have been based on feedback to correct the system behavior. However, instead of being reactive, it's more desirable to be proactive and prevent deviations in the first place from ideal or target value to occur in the response **y**. Prognostics models use feed-forward and develop a functional relationship between input variables and adjust the input variables to achieve the desired results.

In prognostics the intent is to understand the underlying causes of error (variation or uncertainty based on empirical, incompleteness, ambiguity, fuzziness, vagueness, etc.) as much as possible. One can decompose disturbance *d* further to sub-components, namely to disturbances due to other factors (call it *Z*). Thus disturbance *d* can be represented by two variables: a part that can be measured and understood, let's call it *Z*, and by *e* which is the remaining error and unknown cause of variation on output *y*. This is illustrated in Figure 8.4. Thus, now the error term can be written as:

$$d = \{e\ , Z\} \tag{9}$$

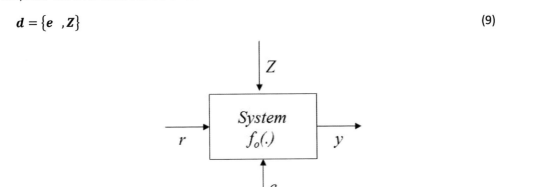

Fig. 8.4 - System with decomposition of error d into e and Z

When the system is shown with prognostics P and prediction Z, one can introduce an intervention process to modify the input u into the system as shown in Figure 8.5.

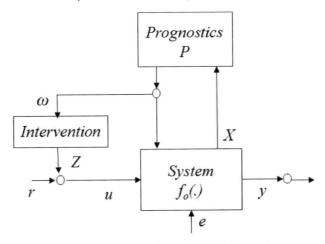

Figure 2.5 - Prognostics P with feed-forward ω

Therefore, the entire disturbance can be explained and measured partly by *Z* and by the remaining disturbance or error represented by *e*. One can measure this disturbance *Z* (though it's not possible to change or control disturbance) to determine how to change the input variables to create feed-forward and maintain the system response variable *y* closer to the target. In this model, *X* is the measured data collected from the system by monitoring certain internal variables.

The goal is to expand on this notion by including the role of three additional components; Monitoring, Memory and Intervention modules in this feed-forward model. In Figure 9, a process for monitoring and collecting measurement data is shown that's represented by **X**, and obtained from the system. The goal of the Prognostics engine is to determine **Z** based on data collected by the monitoring module and prior historical data collected in a memory module. The prognostics engine applies logic to both the measured and historical data represented by **h**, to determine **Z**. The memory module is passive as it stores historical data and provides that data upon recall by the Prognostics engine.

The monitoring module is subject to noise represented by **n**. The input value to the System is represented by **u** as shown in Figure 8.6.

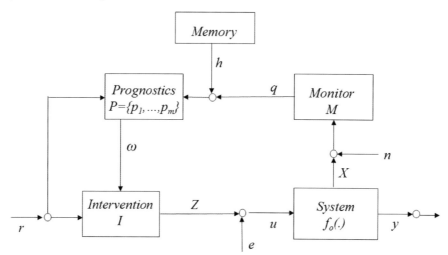

Fig. 8.6: Feed-forward process with Monitor, Prognostics, Memory and Intervention

The input-output signals have the following interpretations:

r   reference or command input

u   System input

e   External disturbance

y   System output

X   Set of monitored and measured signal collected

n   Sensor noise

q   Measured signal, input to Prognostics engine

h   Historical measurements

Z   Prognostics output

P   Set of Prognostics rules

The three signals coming from outside- **r**, **n** and **e** –are known as exogenous inputs.

In the model above, we're interested in well-posedness, namely all transfer functions exist and produce the outputs from the three exogenous inputs.

Next, consider a feed-forward-feedback control model, by taking the output signal through a controller (or observer) and feed it back into the input. This model is shown in Figure 10. An observer process converts the output into signal **v** and feeds it back to an operator that either adds or subtracts from the input signal.

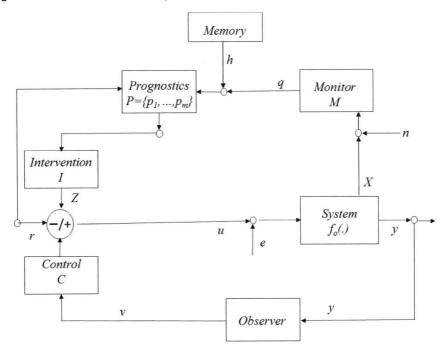

Fig. 8.7 - Combined Feed-forward and feedback model with input, output signals

8.3 Why Feed-forward Control?

There are two potential issues associated with feedback control: First, the time lag to receive the output back into the controller is often too long and as a result there is insufficient time to correct the input. Second, there are situations where the rate of change in disturbance and deviation from a target range of output is slight and gradual over a long time. Finding the exact correction value to the input in order to cancel the disturbance in such systems can be difficult. In several systems, including human health system these conditions can be present where either the onset of an ailment is sudden which does not afford adequate time to respond, or the patient's health decay are too gradual to notice until a sudden change occurs.

Feed-forward control on the other hand offers the ability to apply corrections before the system output falls out of the desired range. Combining feed-forward plus feedback control provides significant improvement over feedback control.

The result of timely prediction and intervention enables physicians to reduce the occurrence of medical complications such as DVT through prevention. For illustration refer to the conceptual graphs in Figure 8.8. Graph (a) represents a conceptual frequency of DVT cases that occur without predictive tools. In contrast, graph (b) represents a smaller and delayed frequency of cases as a result of earlier prediction and intervention.

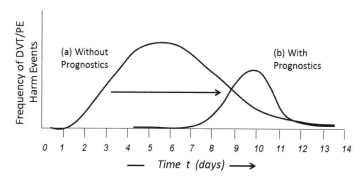

Fig. 8.8 - Harm event distribution graphs with and without prognostics

8.4 Why Artificial Neural Network Algorithms

Of the various statistical and computational methods covered in predictive medical models, Artificial Neural Networks offer unique advantages that make them a suitable tool for research and prognostics. These advantages outweigh some of the criticisms that have been leveled against ANNs (TU 1996).

The primary criticisms of ANNs include a "black-box" approach to data, proneness to over-fitting and greater computational burden. Requiring greater computational power is less of an issue now as the desk top and portable computers have much more powerful computational power. The criticism about "black-box" approach is not a serious limitation in this framework since multiple models are used and supervised learning is applied. Over-fitting is a weakness that occurs when a model is trained to a specific data set and performs poorly on other datasets not used in training. This weakness can be avoided through multiple iterations of cross-validation and setting aside a separate test data batch as employed in this framework. Additionally using multiple models can overcome the issue of one model getting over-trained by one data set versus another data set.

In contrast the advantages and reasons for choosing ANNs as predictive models are significant considerations:

- Ability to model complex non-linear relationships between input data and output
- Ability to learn and adapt to patterns in data
- Resilience towards missing data elements
- Many algorithms are available to choose from
- Ability to handle a large amount of variables
- Ability to handle diverse types of data
- Ability to detect all possible interactions among predictor variables

8.5 Introduction to ANNs

This study applied and compared prediction results from all four neural network models. Neural networks have been successfully applied to classify patterns based on learning from prior examples. Different neural network models use different learning rules, but in general they determine pattern statistics from a set of training examples and then classify new data according to the trained rules. Stated differently, a trained neural network model classifies (or maps) a set of input data to a specific disease from a set of diseases.

Artificial Neural Networks (ANNs) are inspired by the biological learning processes. ANN models are parallel information processing constructs that attempt to mimic certain biological neural systems. ANN offer many advantages: they can model both linear and non-linear problems. They can scale up and down depending on the size. Their parallel construct provides self-healing and redundancy. Models based on ANN constructs attempt to answer several questions about learning, classification and pattern recognition. These attributes are useful features of cognitive and reasoning that occur in medical decision making.

The goal of ANN is to mimic the nervous system. Just as the nervous system consists of an interconnection of simple units, called nerve cells, an ANN consists of many independent but inter-related elements (called neurons) organized into layers. Each neuron transmits an excitation or inhibitory signal to another neuron. The contribution of the signals depends on the strength of the synaptic connection. Similarly, biological neural learning happens by the modification of the synaptic strength. In a neural network the synaptic strengths are represented by weights associated with each input.

A typical ANN is composed of layers connected to each other by full or random connections. There are typically two layers with connection to the external world: an input layer where data is collected and an output layer that presents the outcome or response of the network. But multi-layer ANN models are common. Figure 8.9 shows the a simple neuron consisting of input signals designated by $x_1,..., x_k$, weights associated with each signal $w_{i1},..., w_{ik}$, a summing junction and an activation function that produces output Y_i.

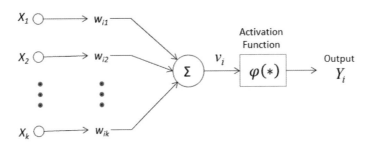

Fig. 8.9 - A simple Neuron with activation function for node i

For each neuron, the summation function aggregates a weighted sum of inputs while the activation function transforms the sum into the final output of the neuron. The formula of each step is shown below:

$$v_i = \sum_{j=1}^{k} x_j w_{ij} \qquad (10)$$

$$Y_i = \varphi(*) \qquad (11)$$

In Figure 8.10 the general structure of a multi-layer ANN is shown. The data gathered about a patient's condition is fed into the model through a layer of neurons. Here four input signals are shown. The result of each layer is an activation function whose output is input to the next layer. There are *m* rules in the framework, each detecting a particular disease. Layers are shown by neurons q_{jpm} and weights that connect layer *(p+1)* to layer *p* by w_{ijpm}, where *i* denotes the number of neuron in layer *p* and *j* the number of neuron in layer *(p+1)*; the subscript *m* denotes the perceptron parameters for model *m*.

157

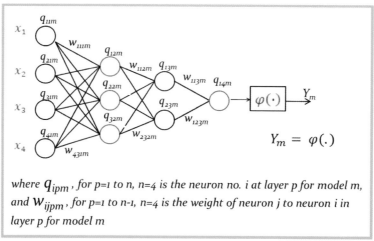

where q_{ipm}, for p=1 to n, n=4 is the neuron no. i at layer p for model m, and W_{ijpm}, for p=1 to n-1, n=4 is the weight of neuron j to neuron i in layer p for model m

Fig. 8.10 - A 4-layer Neural Network

Then the equation to calculate the value of every neuron in each layer in the *n*-layer network above can be described as:

$$q_{i(p+1)m} = \sum_{j=1}^{k-p+1} q_{jpm} W_{ijpm}, \text{ for } p=1, \dots, n\text{-}1, \text{ and layers, } i=1, \dots, k\text{-}p \qquad (12)$$

where *k* is the number of input measurements *x(t)*. Some well-known documented advantages of ANN are learning and pattern recognition. Depending on the activation function, the final output can be a "1" or "0" indicating whether the patient is in danger of developing DVT/PE symptoms or not. Among the training methods, Back-propagation is a common technique for training neural networks. This framework used this technique to train a model and applied it to new set of patient data for predictive purposes.

Back-propagation consists of two steps: In step one; the researcher calculates error contributions to the response function *Y*. This step computes how much each neuron has contributed to the total error in the response value. Error is defined as the difference between the ideal (or expected) result versus the actual response value. Neurons with higher weights have contributed more to the total error and therefore their weight needs to be adjusted more. In step two, the algorithm adjusts the weights starting from the outer layer neurons going back to the hidden layers finally reaching the weights of the input layer. When this algorithm completes, the network has been trained. This is called supervised learning because it defines the ideal (or expected) response value.

Once the neural network model is trained, it can be applied to a fresh or incomplete set of data. The outputs will provide predictions based on the inputs and adjusted weights.

8.6 A Simple Example

The following are two examples of simple, single-layer perceptron classification. These examples are adapted to this framework. The original examples appear in Zurada (Zurada 1997), Haykin (Haykin 1998), Sengupta (Sengupta 2009), and Masters (Masters 1995). One can classify input data about patients into two categories of predictions: DVT-True and DVT-False, by looking at prior patient data. The objective of the single-layer perceptron is to determine a linear boundary that classifies the patients on either side of the linear boundary. As shown in Figure 8.11, the intent is to classify patients into two categories separating by a boundary called a decision boundary line. A linear set of equations define this boundary. The region where the linear equation is >0 is one class (DVT-True), and the region where the linear equation is <0 is the other class (DVT-False). The line is defined as:

$$w_1 x_1 + w_2 x_2 + w_0 = 0$$

One can apply a threshold function to classify patients based on the following threshold function:

$$p(x_1, x_2) = \begin{cases} 1 & if\ w_1 x_1 + w_2 x_2 + w_0 \geq 0 \\ -1 & if\ w_1 x_1 + w_2 x_2 + w_0 < 0 \end{cases}$$

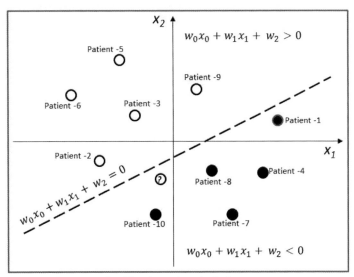

Fig. 8.11 - Classification using single-layer perceptron

Suppose we're considering classifying patients by only four input variables, Glucose (G), Body mass (M), Systolic Blood pressure (S) and White blood cell count (B), represented by x_1, x_2, x_3, and x_4. The threshold function would be computed as follows:

$$p(x_1, x_2, x_3, x_4) = \begin{cases} 1 & if\ w_0 + \sum_{i=1}^{4} w_i x_i\ \geq 0 \\ -1 & if\ w_0 + \sum_{i=1}^{4} w_i x_i\ \leq 0 \end{cases}$$

Let's assume the following weights and input values for classification example are given as shown in Table 1. We can assume the disease under study is DVT.

Table 8.1: Computing classification using single layer perceptron classification

Weights	Values	Inputs	Values
w_1	2	x_1	-1
w_2	0	x_2	2
w_3	3	x_3	0
w_4	-1	x_4	-4
w_0	1	Bias	1
$p(x_1, x_2, x_3, x_4) =$ 2*-1 + 0*2 + 3*0 + -1*-4 + 1*1 = 3			

$\Rightarrow$ class = 1 or DVT-True

If this classification is incorrect, then it's necessary to adjust the weights and repeat the process until the patient is correctly classified. Suppose the correct classification is (-1), then the calculation proceeds as shown in Table 2. The results indicate which class the data belongs to, which in this example the classification is no-disease or DVT-False.

Table 8.2: Revising weights to correct misclassification

Weights	Values	Inputs	Values	New Weight calculation when actual class = -1
w_1	2	x_1	-1	$w_1 = w_1 + class * x_1 = 2 + (-1) * (-1) = 3$
w_2	0	x_2	2	$w_2 = w_2 + class * x_2 = 0 + (-1) * 2 = -2$
w_3	3	x_3	0	$w_3 = w_3 + class * x_3 = 3 + (-1) * 0 = 3$
w_4	-1	x_4	-4	$w_4 = w_4 + class * x_4 = -1 + (-1) * (-4) = 3$
w_0	1	Bias	1	$w_0 = w_0 + class * x_0 = 1 + (-1) * 1 = 0$
$p(x_1, x_2, x_3, x_4) =$ 3*-1 + -2*2 + 3*0 + -1*3 + 0*1 = -7 $\Rightarrow$ class = -1 or DVT-False					

8.7 A Simplified Mathematical Example

In this section, a simple ANN model is presented as an example using the XOR logic table for illustration. As shown in Table 3, the XOR table returns value of 0 if both inputs are identical (both 0's or 1's) and returns value of 1 if one or the other input is a 1.

Table 3: The XOR Logic Table and Results from ANN Model

Input x_1	Input x_2	Ideal Value
0	0	0
0	1	1
1	0	1
1	1	0

It's possible to develop a 3-layer neural network to compute the result for each pair of inputs x_1 and x_2. A third input called Bias is also introduced to construct the model. The value of Bias is always 1. In the first iteration random weights are used. There are a total of 9 weights in this model as shown in Figure 8.12. Simply put, the output is a function of weights and inputs. This is an example of supervised learning as the weights in the ANN model get trained to produce the desired output.

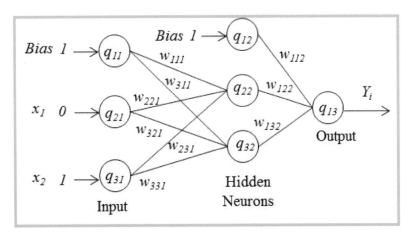

Fig. 8.12 - A 3-layer ANN Network to Compute the XOR Logic Table

The goal is to adjust the weights iteratively until the ANN model produces the Ideal Value. In the first iteration, the model produces some results shown in the Output column. The model computes the error as Mean Square Error (MSE) and uses the error to adjust the weights. The iterations continue and weights get adjusted until the error term is below a threshold (in this case less than 0.009). Eventually the ANN model stops and the output is the Final result as shown in the last column in Table 4. The computed results are close to the ideal values (close to 0 or 1), only different by a small margin of error.

Table8.4: The XOR Logic Table and Results from ANN Model

Input x_1	Input x_2	Ideal Value	Output	$(Error)^2$	Final Results
0	0	0	0.2	0.04	.00875
0	1	1	0.3	0.49	.99130
1	0	1	0.4	0.36	.99123
1	1	0	0.5	0.25	.00568

8.8 Activation Functions

One of the key features of Artificial Neural Networks is that one can map a linear neuron output into a non-linear activation function (Haykin 1998, Sengupta 2009, Zurada 1997). Given inputs $x_0, x_1, ..., x_n$, the output v_k is the result of summation from Equation (10) and $Y_k = \varphi(*)$ is the result of the activation function. The activation function results in an S-shaped curve known as the sigmoid function. There are three types of activation functions. In the first type, as v_k changes from $-\infty$ to $+\infty$, the output can vary from 0 to 1, namely $y_k = [0,1]$. This is the logistics function shown in Figure 8.13. The activation function for this type of neural network is shown as:

$$\varphi(*) = \frac{1}{1 + \exp(-av)} \tag{13}$$

$$\varphi(*) = \begin{cases} 1 & when\ v \to +\infty \\ 0 & when\ v \to -\infty \end{cases} \tag{14}$$

This is the simplest neuron formulation. It's possible to change the shape of the S-curve by changing the values of a. When a is small, the curve appears as smooth function. But, when a is very large, this function

161

approaches the threshold function, a model proposed by Pitts and McCollough (It's also known as the Pitts-McCollough model).

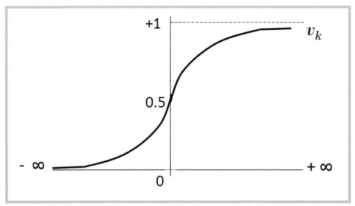

Figure 3 Sigmoid function for activation function v_k between [0,1]

The second type of activation function has a range from -1 to +1, shown with the following equation:

$$\varphi(v) = \tanh(av) \qquad (15)$$

The tanh(.) is the hyperbolic tangent function computed as follows:

$$\tanh(v) = \frac{e^v - e^{-v}}{e^v + e^{-v}} \qquad (16)$$

The activation function $\varphi(v)$ is determined according to the value of v:

$$\varphi(*) = \begin{cases} 1 & when\ v \to +\infty \\ -1 & when\ v \to -\infty \end{cases} \qquad (17)$$

The shape of S-curve representing this activation function is shown in Figure 8.14.

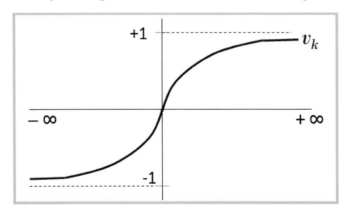

Fig. 8.14 - Activation function for v_k between [-1, 1]

The third type of activation function is the stochastic model determined by:

$$\varphi(v) = \begin{cases} 1 & with\ prob\ p(v) \\ 0 & with\ prob\ 1 - p(v) \end{cases} \qquad (18)$$

162

and $p(v) = \dfrac{1}{1+e^{(-v/T)}}$ $\hspace{6cm}$ (19)

When $p(v) = 1$ then $T = 0$ and this activation function becomes a deterministic model. As T gets larger, there is more stochastic behavior in the model. To better illustrate the role of T, it's possible to think of it as temperature or kinetic energy borrowing this concept loosely from the third law of thermodynamics. Figure 8.15 shows the S-curve associated with this activation function. The various S-curves illustrate the effect of T on the values on the curve.

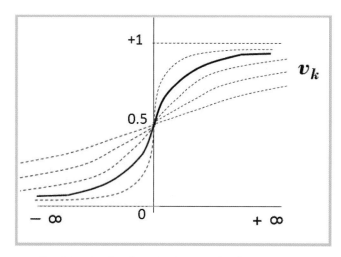

Fig. 8.15 - Stochastic Activation Function for v_k

8.9 Mathematical Foundations of Artificial Neural Networks

A mathematical foundation of ANNs is presented in this section using the common conventions of ANN formulations, so inputs are represented by x, the desired output by d, weights by w, and ANN's output by y (Zurada 1997, Haykin 1998, Wang 2012, Sengupta 2009). As introduction a simple neuron is presented followed by formulations for classification, memory and learning. A single neuron can be constructed with a single activation function. Consider finding a regression line for the histogram shown in Figure 8.16. The regression line is represented by

$y = mx + b$ $\hspace{8cm}$ (20)

Where m is the slope of the line and b is a constant, known as bias. The corresponding neural network representation uses a single neuron where weight parameter w_{11} corresponds to slope m and w_{10} is equal to a constant 1.0.

163

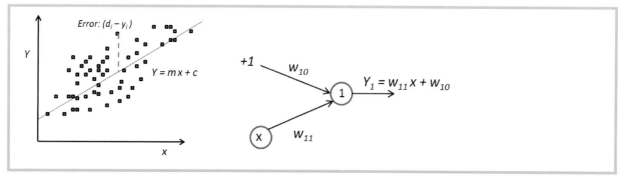

Fig. 8.16 - A regression line and its equivalent single neuron representation

If y is dependent on multiple inputs x_j, one can think of bias as another input to the neuron with a weight w_{k0}. To find the best fitting line, the goal is to minimize the errors E, by adjusting weights. Given multiple x_j one can use the gradient descent method to find the minimum E and the corresponding weights.

8.10 Gradient Descent Methods

The Gradient Descent method is used as an iterative process to determine the weights associated with each input x. This method which is also known as Error Correction learning in ANN literature works to minimize the total error as the method of training the model and determining the appropriate weights. The following derivation is adapted from Zurada (Zurada 1997) and Sengupta (Sengupta 2009), improved and revised specific to this framework. Total error E can be written as:

$$Total\ Error\ E = \sum_j E_j = \frac{1}{2}\sum_j (d_j - y_j)^2 \qquad (21)$$

This represents the total error E for point j. The expression d_j is the target output (desired output) at point j, and y_j is the actual output at point j.

Let's now consider all possible outputs $y_0, ..., y_m$ where $0 \leq j \leq m$, and

$$y_0 = f_0(x_1, x_2, ..., x_n) \qquad (22)$$

$$y_1 = f_1(x_1, x_2, ..., x_n)$$

...

$$y_m = f_m(x_1, x_2, ..., x_n)$$

Total error E is the combined error of all errors for outputs y_k. It's common to use ½ of the sum in (14) since as will be explained later it makes mathematical manipulations easier as one takes derivative of this term and the gradient will be multiplied by 2.

Let's define the gradient, namely the rate of increase for (i,j) pair connection as:

$$G = \frac{\partial E}{\partial w_{ij}} = \frac{\partial}{\partial w_{ij}} \sum E_j = \sum_j \frac{\partial E_j}{\partial w_{ij}} \qquad (23)$$

Next, it's possible to apply partial derivatives and chain rule to get the following:

$$\frac{\partial E}{\partial w_{ij}} = \frac{\partial E}{\partial y_j} \cdot \frac{\partial y_j}{\partial w_{ij}}$$ (24)

For sake of simplicity let's denote d_j and y_j as follows:

$$d_j = \sum d_j \text{ , and } y_j = \sum y_j$$

One can take derivative of the total Error, Equation (21) to get the following:

$$\frac{\partial E}{\partial y_j} = -(d_j - y_j)$$ (25)

$$y_j = \sum_j w_{ij} x_j$$ (26)

$$\frac{\partial y_0}{\partial w_{oi}} = \frac{\partial}{\partial w_{oi}} \sum_j w_{oj} x_j = x_i$$ (27)

$$\frac{\partial E}{\partial w_{ij}} = -(d_j - y_j)x_i$$ (28)

Where j is the output unit, and i is the input unit. Thus the derivative of error with respect to w_{ij} has been formulated. In order to move the opposite direction to the derivative one can apply the corrections to the w_{ij}'s by multiplying a (-) sign to the difference. The (-) sign is applied because the goal is to minimize error. The correction can be written as:

$$\Delta w_{ij} = (d_j - y_j)x_i$$ (29)

The new synaptic weight will be computed using the following for several iterations until Δw_{ij} is less than a given threshold set by the user:

$$w_{ij\,(new)} = w_{ij\,(old)} + \Delta w_{ij}$$ (30)

It's possible to use η to represent the rate of descent in (29). So η is the learning rate that reduces total error E, with every iteration and can be defined by the researcher to regulate Δw_{ij}, the rate of descent.

8.11 Neural Network Learning Processes

There are five major categories of learning models in Neural Networks. One of these learning methods called Error Correction based learning was already discussed in section 3.2.1. In this section, four other categories are presented that are most relevant to this framework: Memory based learning, Hebbian based learning, Competitive learning and Boltzman learning model. These learning methods are adapted from Sengupta (Sengupta 2009), Zeruda (Zeruda 1997), Wang (Wang 2012), Masters (Masters 1995) and Haykin (Haykin 1998). They're refined and revised for this framework and are included for the sake of completeness.

Memory Based Learning

Memory based learning works to retain relationship between input vector and output. Given input vector $\vec{x}$ defined by $\{x\}_{i=1}^{N}$, and desired output d_i, this association can be shown by the expression $\{x_i, d_i\}_{i=1}^{N}$. When the model is applied to a new pattern $\vec{x}_i$, since this pattern is initially unknown let's start with a test pattern $\vec{x}_{test}$ and find the Euclidean distance between $\vec{x}_{test}$ vector and the new pattern $\vec{x}_i$ vector. Let's assume that $\vec{x}_N' \in \{x_1, x_2, x_3, \dots, x_N\}$ is the set of nearest neighbor points of $\vec{x}_{test}$ vector, then it implies that the distance of pattern $\vec{x}_i$ from $\vec{x}_{test}$ is minimum over the set of all $\vec{x}_i$. This can be shown by the following expression to be true for all distances over i:

$$\min_{(over\ i)} \ d\{x_i, \vec{x}_{test}\} = d(\vec{x}'_N, \vec{x}_{test}) \tag{31}$$

To improve this algorithm it's prudent to look at the nearest neighbors and find the set that offers minimum distances. Memory based learning is ideal for pattern recognition and classification of data as shown by example in Figure 8.17. This approach helps keep outliers out of classification. This is the k-nearest neighbor classification. In Figure 8.17, a point x_i is being classified between the "+" or the "O" shapes. Since its nearest neighbors are the "O" shapes, it will get classified as a member of the "O" set.

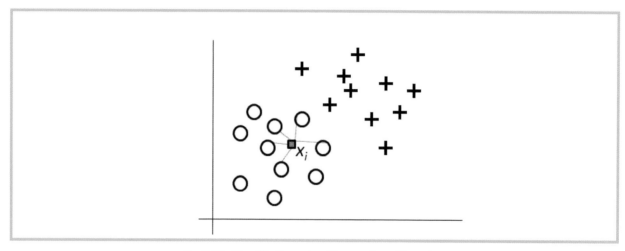

Fig. 8.17 - Classification using Memory Based Learning

Hebbian Based Learning

The goal of the Hebbian based learning is to retain the association between the input vector and the output. This method is attributed to Donald Hebb, a neurobiologist who in 1949 introduced his theories of neuron adaptation in the brain during the learning process. In the Hebbian learning process the amount of adjustment to weight w_{kj} is defined by:

$$\Delta w_{kj}(n) = f(y_k(n), x_j(n)) \tag{32}$$

This is the adjustment in w_{kj} at time step n, as a function of responses y_k and input x_j at time step n. One can re-write this expression in terms of pre-and post-synaptic responses:

$$\Delta w_{kj} = \eta\, y_k(n)\, x_j(n), \tag{33}$$

where η is the rate of learning. This expression is known as the Activity Product Rule. It's important to note that η is constant. Assuming that one keeps x_j constant then it's possible to plot Δw_{kj} and $y_k(n)$ to get a line that intercepts through the origin with slope of $\eta\, x_j(n)$ as shown Figure 8.18. As y_k increases, so does Δw_{kj}. Eventually the synaptic weight reaches its saturation point where not more learning possible.

166

Let's define $\bar{x}$ and $\bar{y}$ as time averaged values of x_j and y_k. Then it's possible to define:

$x_j(n) = x_j - \bar{x}$, and $y_k(n) = y_k - \bar{y}$.

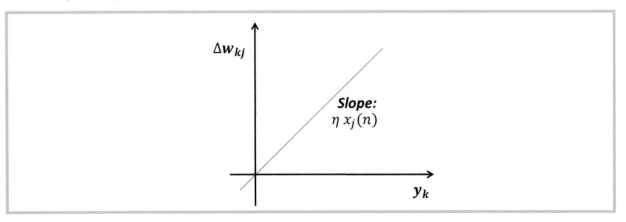

Fig. 8.18 - Slope of Activity Product Rule as rate of learning

By definition of covariance, it's possible to write the change in weights w_{kj} as the covariance of distance of x_j and y_k from their respective time averaged values $\bar{x}$ and $\bar{y}$.

$$\Delta w_{kj} = \eta\,(x_j - \bar{x})(y_k - \bar{y}) \tag{34}$$

Since the average effect of change over the entire input values of x_j is desired, one can recognize $\bar{x}$ as a constant over the course of x_j. This relationship can be shown by a line that intersects Δw_{kj} and y_k as shown in Figure 8.19. This figure shows the relationship between Δw_{kj} and y_k for a given point x_j such that $(x_j - \bar{x})$ is a constant.

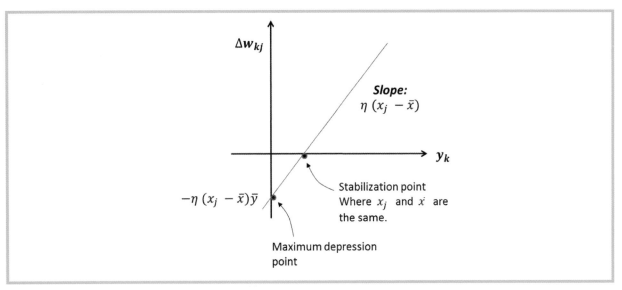

Fig. 8.19 - The covariance relationship between response and input

Using covariance approach, three conditions are possible:

(i) w_{kj} increases if $x_j > \bar{x}$ and $y_k > \bar{y}$

(ii) w_{kj} decreases if either $\begin{cases} a) \; x_j < \bar{x} \; and \; y_k > \bar{y} \\ b) \; x_j > \bar{x} \; and \; y_k < \bar{y} \end{cases}$ (35)

(iii) w_{kj} increases if $x_j < \bar{x}$ and $y_k < \bar{y}$

Competitive Learning

In Competitive learning, each neuron competes to increase its response value while minimizing the other neuron's output. The wining neuron will be preferred in future iterations of learning. The mathematical model of competitive learning is based on:

$$y_k \begin{cases} 1 \; if \; v_k > v_j \,, \; for \; all \; j \; when \; j \neq k. \\ \quad\quad 0 \; otherwise \end{cases}$$ (36)

The sum total of all weights are set to 1 for all k:

$$\sum_j w_{kj} = 1,$$

For example, consider three clusters of input variables as shown in Figure 8.20. One can write x_j as a vector $\vec{x} = [x_1, x_2, \, x_3]$. If the relationship $\|\vec{x}\| = 1$ is enforced, namely that if it's required that $\sqrt{x_1^2 + x_2^2 + x_3^2} = 1$, then there can be several vectors $\vec{x}_1, \vec{x}_2, \vec{x}_3$ to represent different patterns as shown in Figure 8.20. The goal is to classify data into any one of n patterns. The clusters of patterns are grouped into set of data in vectors (in this example in vectors $\vec{x}_1, \vec{x}_2, \vec{x}_3$) such that: $\sum_j w_{kj} = 1$, for all k. In addition, it's possible to show weights for each cluster as a vector. For example, the vector of weights for the first cluster can be shown as: $\vec{w}_1 = [w_{11} \quad w_{12} \quad w_{13}]$.

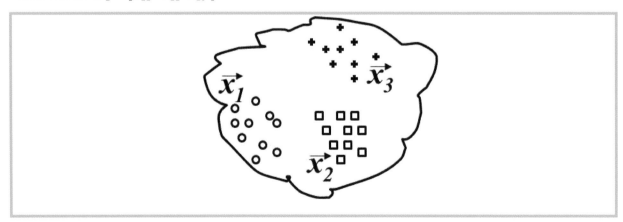

Fig. 8.20 - Using competitive learning to classify data into different patterns

In this competitive learning model, typically the most central element (or neuron) in a cluster is the winner and all other weights conform (or align) to it. The competitive learning rule is that Δw_{kj} is determined by:

$$\Delta w_{kj} = \begin{cases} \eta \left(x_j - w_{kj} \right) & \text{if neuron } k \text{ wins the competition} \\ 0 & \text{if neuron } k \text{ loses} \end{cases}$$

Boltzman Learning Model

The Boltzman learning process is derived from statistical mechanics and mimics a stochastic learning model. In this model the neurons constitute a recurrent structure that allows self-feedback. The neurons take a binary value of +1 or -1. The model is represented by:

$$E = -\frac{1}{2} \sum_j \sum_k w_{kj} x_k x_j \quad \text{where } j \neq k$$

The visible neurons are output layer. The inner neurons as shown in Figure 8.21 are hidden neurons. This model is regarded stochastic as a change in one outer neuron changes the value of E. The probability that a neuron x_k flips it state from one state to another state is defined by:

$$P\left(x_k \rightarrow -x_k \right) = \frac{1}{1 + \exp\left(\frac{-\Delta E_k}{T} \right)}$$

The change in E_k from a flip is denoted by ΔE_k. If E is be regarded as an energy function, then ΔE_k is the change of energy from a flip of state in a neuron. The variable is the pseudo temperature representing the level of noise or stochasticity. Let's assign two variables:

P_{kj}^+: the correlation between neuron k and neuron j in the clamped condition

P_{kj}^-: the correlation between neuron k and neuron j in the free condition

Then the Boltzman learning rule is defined by:

$$\Delta w_{kj} = \eta \left(P_{kj}^+ - P_{kj}^- \right) \quad \text{where } j \neq k.$$

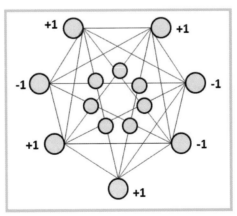

Fig. 8.21 - Inner and Outer Neurons in a Boltzman Learning model

8.12 Selected Analytics models

The appropriate predictive mathematical model must offer accuracy and simplicity to learn from prior cases and easily be extensible to apply new data to make predictions about a patient's health condition. This prediction is possible by classification of a new patient into any one of possible disease categories. Since this framework uses multiple models for classification, it's important that close attention is given to accuracy of each model. The following four models were selected because each provides certain characteristic that make it appropriate for certain type of data and computation. It has also been established that these models are among the most accurate neural network models for classification. Below is a summary of advantages and disadvantages of each ANN method (Masters 1995):

1) PNN - Probabilistic Neural Networks are four layer networks. They classify data in a non-parametric method and are less sensitive to outlier data. It's been demonstrated that probabilistic neural networks using only four layers of input, pattern, summation and output perceptron can provide accurate and relatively faster classifications than the back-propagation neural networks (Principe, Euliano, Lefebvre 1999).

2) SVM – Support Vector Machine networks. SVM performs classification by constructing a two-layer network that defines a hyperplane that separates data into multiple classifications. The SVM is a non-probabilistic binary linear classifier. It takes a set of input data and determines which of possible classes the input is a member of.

3) GFN (Generalized Feed-forward) trained with LM – A feed-forward neural network consists of one or more layers of nodes where the information flows in only one direction, forward from the input nodes and there are no cycles or loops in the network. In the multi-layer model, each node has direct connection to the nodes in the subsequent layer. The sum of products of the weights and the inputs are calculated in each node (Haykin 1999).

4) MLP trained with LM – Multi-layer perceptron, a method similar to gradient descent approach with variable step modification. Several variations of this model have been proposed, including the Levenberg-Marquardt model (Wilamowski & Chen, 1999) which is known to be among the most efficient algorithms.

The next section is a more in-depth mathematical review of the four Neural Network approaches used in this book.

8.13 Probabilistic Neural Networks

Recall the classification problem from Figure 8.22 where the goal is to classify an unknown patient (shown by ?) into one of the two groups. The most straightforward method would be to check the distance from the nearest neighbor. But this method, while simple, has weaknesses. It can be misclassified into one group when in fact it belongs to another groups' cluster. The goal is to define a "sphere of influence" function to represent the spread of distance separating an unknown point from a training set point. Such a function would have a peak at zero distance from the training set point and taper off to zero as the distance increased. A proposed classifier would compute the sum of this function for all training set points of each population and classify the unknown into the population that has the greatest sum.

The following derivation is adapted from Sengupta (Sengupta 2009) and Zurada (Zurada 1997), improved and revised specific to this framework. A mathematical construct that can help define such a function is the Gaussian function:

$$f(x) = ae^{-\frac{(x-x_i)^2}{2\sigma^2}}$$

(37)

Where a, x_i, σ are > 0, and a is the height of the curve's peak (or amplitude), x_i is the position of the center of the peak and σ is the width (or the spread) of the curve. (Hardy 2008) has illustrated a 2-dimensional graph for x_0, x_1 as shown in Figure 8.22, where the values of x_0, x_1 are set to origin (0,0). Coefficients a, and σ can take any positive values.

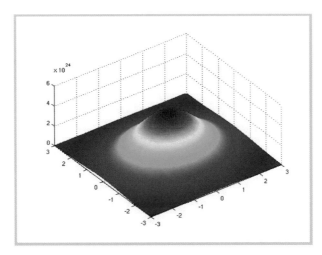

Fig. 8.22 - Graph of a 2-dimenstional Gaussian Function

Using the Gaussian function, (Parzen, 1962) and (Cacoullos, 1966) showed that one can compute the multivariate probability density function from a random sample. Essentially, Parzen's probability density function is a "sphere of influence" function that can be used as the classifier algorithm. The scaling parameter σ controls the width of the area of influence.

The idea behind PNN is that each training element represented by a Gaussian pattern unit, adds to the likelihood that nearby data has the same classification. To compute the classification of a data point, let's calculate the response for the point with every category and select the category that has the highest response. Each trained data point corresponds to pattern unit that is a Gaussian function with its peak centered on the parameter's location. The idea behind this classification approach is that for a new data point, we measure the average "distance" between the new point and all other points in the classification. The smaller the average "distance" of a point to other points results in a larger value of z as computed according to Equation (38). Therefore the point will belong to that classification where its z value is the highest.

Consider a simple Gaussian pattern equation that computes the result for a point (x_0, x_1) relative to already classified points (x_{0i}, x_{1i}):

$$z = f(x_0, x_1) = \sum_{i=1}^{n} e^{\frac{-\left((x_0 - x_{0i})^2 + (x_1 - x_{1i})^2\right)}{2\sigma^2}} \qquad (38)$$

Suppose one intends to predict the future state of a patient's Intra-Cranial Pressure (ICP). The goal is to classify the input data into one of 3 possible classes: Normal, Moderate or Critical. Each class is represented by f_N, f_M and f_C that are probability distribution functions for category N, M and C (Normal, Moderate and Critical). Then one can compute f_N, f_M and f_C as follows:

$$z_N = f_N(x_0, x_1) = \sum_{i=1}^{n} e^{\frac{-\left((x-x_{0Ni})^2 + (x-x_{1Ni})^2\right)}{2\sigma^2}} \tag{39}$$

$$z_M = f_M(x_0, x_1) = \sum_{i=1}^{n} e^{\frac{-\left((x-x_{0Mi})^2 + (x-x_{1Mi})^2\right)}{2\sigma^2}}$$

$$z_C = f_C(x_0, x_1) = \sum_{i=1}^{n} e^{\frac{-\left((x-x_{0Ci})^2 + (x-x_{1Ci})^2\right)}{2\sigma^2}}$$

Here the data point to be classified is x and all the other points that belong to other classifications are referred to by N_i, M_i and C_i. There are many activation functions possible but a common non-linear operation is the following:

$$e^{\frac{-(W_i-X)^t(W_i-X)}{2\sigma^2}} \tag{40}$$

If X and W_i are normalized to unit length, it's been demonstrated (Zaruda 1997) that the non-linear operation above can be replaced by (41). The derivation follows by multiplying the numerator terms that results in:

$$-w_i^2 + 2\,w_i X - X^2 = -2 + 2w_i X = 2(w_i X - 1)$$

Since the terms w_i^2 and X^2 are normalized to unity, they are replaced by 1. Substituting Z_i for $W_i X$ in the above term in the numerator, one can obtain the following activation function:

$$e^{\frac{(Z_i - 1)}{\sigma^2}} \tag{41}$$

So a simple algorithm to identify classification of a new data set can be described as:

1. Input layer: Normalize X and W_i to unit length
2. Pattern layer: Compute the dot product of input X and weights of X, W_i
3. Summation layer: Compute f_N, f_M and f_C
4. Output (or decision) layer: Select output with highest response value (from N, M or C clusters of neurons)

The final classification is determined by a classifier function C that selects the largest of f_N, f_M and f_C values:

$$Prediction_{(t+t1)} = C\,(f_N, f_M, f_C) = max(f_N, f_M, f_C) \tag{42}$$

An Example in Appendix B illustrates how PNN can be applied to a simple classification problem.

8.14 Support Vector Machine (SVM) Networks

Support Vector Machines (SVM) are among supervised training models that analyze data for multiple classification and regression analysis. The SVM is a no-probabilistic binary linear classifier. It takes a set of input data and determines which of possible classes the input is a member of. SVM constructs a set of hyperplanes between data elements to classify them. A good separation is the mark of a generalizable model and is achieved by the hyperplane that has the largest distance to the nearest training data element in any class. The hyperplane is mathematically defined as the set of data elements whose inner product with a vector in that space is constant. Margin is the distance between the optimal hyperplane and a vector that runs close to it.

The following derivation is adapted from Sengupta (Sengupta 2009) and Haykin (Haykin 1998), improved and revised specific to this framework.

The most optimum solution can be found by gaining the biggest possible margin. The optimal hyperplane must satisfy:

$$\frac{y_k F(x_k)}{||w||} \geq \tau, \ k = 1, 2, \dots, n \tag{43}$$

where τ is the margin and can be visualized as a band that separates the nears points from the hyperplane that separates them into two categories Note that F(x) is defined by:

$$F(x) = w^T x + b \tag{44}$$

One can map the data points to a very high-dimensional space, then the algorithm finds a hyperplane in this space with the largest margin separating classes of data. The feature space is usually defined as a non-linear product of base functions $\varphi_i(x)$, defined in the input space. Then function *F(x)* becomes:

$$F(x) = \sum_{i=1}^{n} a_i K(x_i, x) + b \tag{45}$$

where $K(x_i, x)$ is the inner product kernel of base functions $\varphi_i(x), j = 1, 2, \dots, m$. The cross products in the larger space are defined by a kernel function *K(x, y)* that best fits the problem, such that:

$$\sum_i a_i K(x_i, x) = constant \tag{46}$$

It can observed that *K(x,y)* becomes small as *y* grows further from x. The inner product K(.) can have many possible kernels, one of the most commonly used is based on the Gaussian:

$$K(x_i, x) = e^{\left(-\frac{||x - x_i||^2}{2\sigma^2}\right)} \tag{47}$$

where $\sigma > 0$, and sigmoid kernels

$$K(x_i, x) = \tanh(\theta < x_i, \ x > + \vartheta) \qquad \text{such that } \theta > 0, \ and \ x > + \vartheta. \tag{48}$$

8.15 General Feed-forward Neural Network

A feed-forward neural network consists of one or more layers of nodes where the information flows in only one direction, forward from the input nodes and there are no cycles or loops in the network. The simplest networks have single layer that feeds input data to the output layer via a series of weights. One of the popular training methods is the Gradient Descent algorithm. The following is a mathematical development of the Gradient descent method, adapted from Sengupta (Sengupta 2009) and Zurada (Zurada 1997) and improved for this framework.

For a given neural network with *n=1,...,N* layers, one can compute the error for each node. By definition the error at time snapshot *n,* for node *j* computed by:

$$e_j(n) = d_j(n) - y_j(n) \tag{49}$$

And for computing total error of a network, recall Equation (21) provides that:

$$E(n) = \frac{1}{2} \sum_j e_j^2(n) \qquad \text{for } j=1 \text{ to } m. \tag{50}$$

Then one can compute average error of a network by:

$$E(N)_{Avg} = \frac{1}{N} \sum_{n=1}^{N} E(n) \tag{51}$$

Let's use the traditional Pitts-McCullough equation to compute:

$$v_j(n) = \sum_{i=0}^{m} w_{ji}(n) y_i(n) , \tag{52}$$

where $v_j(n)$ is the input to activation function for the neuron j. The term $v_j(n)$ can be perceived as the induced local field while $y_j(n)$ can be thought of as the output from the previous layer, shown by:

$$y_j(n) = \varphi(v_j(n)) \tag{53}$$

Given the prior introduction, it's possible to start the mathematical derivation of back-propagation method. First it's easy to calculate the partial derivative of $E(n)$ and apply the chain rule to obtain the following:

$$\frac{\partial E(n)}{\partial w_{ji}(n)} = \frac{\partial E(n)}{\partial e_j(n)} \cdot \frac{\partial e_j(n)}{\partial y_j(n)} \cdot \frac{\partial y_j(n)}{\partial v_j(n)} \cdot \frac{\partial v_j(n)}{\partial w_{ji}(n)} \tag{54}$$

Where Δw_{ji} is applied to w_{ji}. Let's apply the derivatives to each component above:

$$\frac{\partial E(n)}{\partial e_j(n)} = e_j(n)$$

$$\frac{\partial e_j(n)}{\partial y_j(n)} = -1$$

$$\frac{\partial y_j(n)}{\partial v_j(n)} = \varphi'(v_j(n)), \text{ and one can take derivative of } \varphi(v_j(n)) \text{ when the exact function is known.}$$

$$\frac{\partial v_j(n)}{\partial w_{ji}(n)} = y_i(n)$$

Now it's possible to write the result of substitutions as:

$$\frac{\partial E(n)}{\partial w_{ji}(n)} = - e_j(n) \, \varphi'(v_j(n)) \, y_i(n) \tag{55}$$

When adjustment of $\Delta w_{ji}(n)$ (namely the correction to $w_{ji}(n)$ is applied to $w_{ji}(n)$ the following relationship can be obtained:

$$\Delta w_{ji}(n) = -\eta \frac{\partial E(n)}{\partial w_{ji}(n)} = \eta \, e_j(n) \, \varphi'(v_j(n)) \, y_i(n) \tag{56}$$

This equation is a reminder that $\Delta w_{ji}(n)$ is proportional to $\frac{\partial E(n)}{\partial w_{ji}(n)}$ at a rate of proportionality η, negative to the direction of the gradient. Part of the term in (55) can be described as error multiplied by activation function. This term can be shown as:

$$\partial_j(n) = - \frac{\partial E(n)}{\partial v_j(n)} = - \frac{\partial E(n)}{\partial e_j(n)} \cdot \frac{\partial e_j(n)}{\partial y_j(n)} \cdot \frac{\partial y_j(n)}{\partial v_j(n)} \tag{57}$$

$$\partial_j(n) = e_j(n) \, \varphi'(v_j(n)) \tag{58}$$

The term $\partial_j(n)$ is the derivative of error with respect to the activation function $v_j(n)$. This is the gradient for neuron j and is local to neuron j. This is also known the local gradient. Now one can rewrite the equation (56) as:

$$\Delta w_{ji}(n) = \eta\, \partial_j(n)\, y_i(n) \quad \text{where } y_i(n) \text{ is the input to neuron } j. \tag{59}$$

Since the values for η and $y_i(n)$ are known it's possible to compute $\partial_j(n)$. Two cases are possible:

Case 1) Neuron j belongs to the output layer, hence $\partial_j(n)$ can be calculated from equation (54).

Case 2) Neuron j belongs to a hidden layer, thus $\partial_j(n)$ must be computed differently.

A fundamental condition for back-propagation is that one can compute $\partial_j(n)$, namely the derivative of the activation function is possible. Let's examine this approach graphically to illustrate the hidden layer and output layer computations as shown in Figure 8.23. The signal flow graph in Figure 8.23 shows j is the hidden layer and k as output layer neurons.

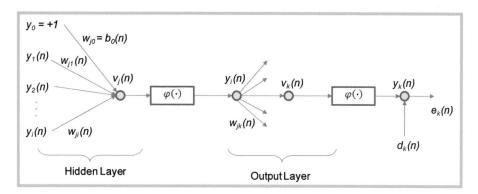

Fig. 8.23 - Depiction of hidden layer j and output layer k neurons

One can compute $\partial_j(n)$ by the following derivations. It's known that:

$$\partial_j(n) = -\frac{\partial E(n)}{\partial v_j(n)} = -\frac{\partial E(n)}{\partial y_j(n)} \cdot \varphi'\big(v_j(n)\big) \tag{60}$$

Also recall from equation (50) that:

$E(n) = \frac{1}{2} \sum_k e_k^2(n)$, where k is the set of output layer neurons. It can be shown that:

$$\frac{\partial E(n)}{\partial y_j(n)} = \sum_k e_k(n)\frac{\partial e_k(n)}{\partial y_j(n)} = \sum_k e_k(n)\frac{\partial e_k(n)}{\partial v_k(n)} \cdot \frac{\partial v_k(n)}{\partial y_j(n)} \tag{61}$$

$$\text{Since } e_j(n) = d_j(n) - y_j(n) = d_j(n) - \varphi(v_j(n)) \tag{62}$$

Let's take derivatives of the left hand side:

$$\frac{\partial e_k(n)}{\partial v_k(n)} = -\varphi'\big(v_k(n)\big) \tag{63}$$

For neuron k, it's possible to write:

$$v_k(n) = \sum_{j=0}^{m} w_{kj}(n) y_j(n) \qquad (64)$$

Consequently by taking derivate of (64), it results in the following:

$$\frac{\partial v_k(n)}{\partial y_i(n)} = w_{kj}(n) \qquad (65)$$

$$\frac{\partial E(n)}{\partial y_j(n)} = -\sum_k e_k(n) \, \varphi'\big(v_k(n)\big) w_{kj}(n) = -\sum_k \partial_j(n) w_{kj}(n) \qquad (66)$$

From equation (60) and (66) one can conclude that:

$$\partial_j(n) = \varphi_j'\big(v_j(n)\big) \cdot \sum_k \partial_k(n) w_{kj}(n) \qquad (67)$$

This equation is significant as it shows that the local gradient of neuron j (hidden neurons) depends on the local gradient of output neuron k. The summation is the weighted sum of all the output gradients. Let's assume M is the number of output neurons. Consider multiplying each error term $e_j(n)$ by the derivative of the corresponding activation function $\varphi_k(v_k(n))$, namely by $\varphi_k'(v_k(n))$. This is the basis of back-propagation as depicted in Figure 8.24.

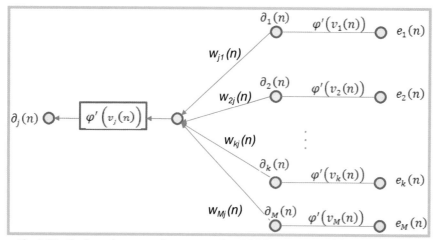

Fig. 8.24 - Backward propagation - computing $\partial_j(n)$ from errors $e_k(n)$ in forward step

In forward pass, the inputs propagate forward from 1st layer to the 2nd layer and so on to eventually to the output layer. The error terms are computed and then the backward propagation begins. In backward propagation, the algorithm starts with the error term. Then it calculates the local gradients and propagate back and adjust the synaptic weights.

Activation function can be any of the three types mentioned previously, such as the sigmoid function, logistic function or a *tanh( )* function. Let's compute the derivative of activation function for the case of the logistic function:

$$\varphi_j\big(v_j(n)\big) = \frac{1}{1 + e^{\left(-av_j(n)\right)}} \equiv y_j(n) \qquad (68)$$

It's given that $a > 0$, and $-\infty < v_j(n) < \infty$. It's possible to compute the derivative of the activation function as follows:

$$\varphi_j'(v_j(n)) = \frac{a \cdot e^{(-av_j(n))}}{[1 + e^{(-av_j(n))}]^2} \qquad = a \cdot y_j(n)[1 - y_j(n)] \tag{69}$$

In other words one can write the above in the following fashion:

$$\varphi_j'(v_j(n)) = [1 - y_j(n)] \cdot (a) \cdot (y_j(n)) \tag{70}$$

Now one can use $y_j(n)$ for computing $\partial_j(n)$ by:

$$\partial_j(n) = \varphi_j'(v_j(n)) \cdot \sum_k \partial_k(n) w_{kj}(n) =$$

$$a \cdot y_j(n)[1 - y_j(n)] \sum_k \partial_k(n) w_{kj}(n) \tag{71}$$

The range of $y_j(n)$ is [0,1]. The value of $\varphi_j'(v_j(n))$ is maximum when $y_j = 0.50$, and $\varphi_j'(v_j(n))$ is equal to zero when $y_j = 1.0$ or zero. This fact guides our choice of proper values for Δw_{kj}. Similarly one could have taken derivative of $tanh(x)$, to compute Δw_{kj}. A detailed description of this algorithm appears in Appendix C.

8.16 MLP with Levenberg-Marquardt (LM) Algorithm

Feed-forward MLP with LM is a feed-forward neural network that consists of one or more layers of nodes where the information flows in only one direction, forward from the input nodes and there are no cycles or loops in the network (Sengupta 2009, Masters 1995). The simplest networks have single layer that feeds input data to the output layer via a series of weights. In the multi-layer perceptron model (MLP), each node has direct connection to the nodes in the subsequent layer. The sum of products of the weights and the inputs are calculated in each node (Haykin 1999). If the value of the result is above a certain threshold, the neuron fires with the activated value (typically 1), otherwise, it fires the deactivated value (typically -1). Several variations of this model and training methods have been proposed, including the backward propagation algorithm and Levenberg-Marquardt (LM) method which is considered as one of the more computationally efficient algorithms. The following derivation is adapted from Sengupta (Sengupta 2009), Haykin (Haykin 1998) and Masters (Masters 1995), revised and improved for this framework.

The training of MLP occurs in two stages: in a forward phase the weights of the network are fixed and the input data is propagated through the network. The forward phase completes its computation with an error signal. The error term was defined by Equation (49) and can be written specifically to can be defined as

$$e_{kp} = d_{kp} - y_{kp}, \quad k = 1, \dots, K, \quad p = 1, \dots, P \tag{72}$$

where d_{kp} is the desired response and y_{kp} is the actual output produced by the network response to the input x_{ip}. d_{kp} is the desired value of the kth output and the Pth layer. Y_{kp} is the actual value of the kth output and P^{th} pattern. The parameter K is the number of network outputs, P is the number of patterns and N is the number of weights.

The backward phase the error e_{kp} is propagated through the network going backward and the free weights are adjusted to minimize error e_{kp}. In the LM algorithm, the performance index $F(W)$ is to be optimized:

$$F(W) = \sum_{p=1}^{P}\left[\sum_{k=1}^{K}(d_{kp} - y_{kp})^2\right] \tag{73}$$

Where $W = [w_1\ w_2\ ...\ w_N]^T$ is the set of all weights for the network. The equation can be written as:

$$F(W) = E^T E$$

$$\text{Where } E = [e_{11}\ ....\ e_{K1}\ e_{12}\ ...\ e_{K2}\ ...\ e_{1P}\ ...\ e_{KP}]^T \tag{74}$$

The error term E, is the cumulative error vector for all patterns. Let's assume that the amount of change to each weight is shown by .Using the Jacobian matrix one can compute the amount of change that be applied to weights in the backward propagation. By definition, a Jacobian is the derivative of one vector with respect to another vector. From the equation above, the Jacobian matrix can be defined as:

$$J = \begin{bmatrix} \dfrac{\partial e_{11}}{\partial w_1} & \dfrac{\partial e_{11}}{\partial w_2} & \cdots & \dfrac{\partial e_{11}}{\partial w_N} \\[2mm] \dfrac{\partial e_{21}}{\partial w_1} & \dfrac{\partial e_{21}}{\partial w_2} & \cdots & \dfrac{\partial e_{21}}{\partial w_N} \\[1mm] \vdots & \vdots & & \vdots \\[1mm] \dfrac{\partial e_{K1}}{\partial w_1} & \dfrac{\partial e_{K1}}{\partial w_1} & & \dfrac{\partial e_{K1}}{\partial w_1} \\[1mm] \vdots & \vdots & & \vdots \\[1mm] \dfrac{\partial e_{1P}}{\partial w_1} & \dfrac{\partial e_{1P}}{\partial w_2} & \cdots & \dfrac{\partial e_{1P}}{\partial w_N} \\[1mm] \dfrac{\partial e_{2P}}{\partial w_1} & \dfrac{\partial e_{2P}}{\partial w_2} & & \dfrac{\partial e_{2P}}{\partial w_N} \\[1mm] \vdots & \vdots & & \vdots \\[1mm] \dfrac{\partial e_{KP}}{\partial w_1} & \dfrac{\partial e_{KP}}{\partial w_2} & & \dfrac{\partial e_{KP}}{\partial w_N} \end{bmatrix} \tag{75}$$

Using the Newton-Raphson method, one can compute the change in weight by applying a dampened measure of error terms. It's possible to derive the Levenberg-Marquardt algorithm as follows. Recall that the output is a function of inputs x_i and weights W. This can be stated by writing:

$$y_i = y_i\,(x_i, W)$$

In other words, y_i depends on input x_i and weights W. The goal of backward propagation is to adjust the weights W by $J_i\delta$ where δ is the amount of adjustment and J_i is the ith row of the Jacobian matrix. Then it's possible to write this expression as:

$$y_i(x_i, W + \delta) \cong y_i\,(x_i, W) + J_i\delta$$

The goal of computation is to minimize the objective function in Equation (73):

Minimize $E(W) = \sum_p \sum_k (d_i - y_i)^2$

When adjusted by δ, the minimization function can be written as:

$$E(W + \delta) = \sum_p \sum_k (d_i - y_i(x_i, W + \delta))^2 \cong \sum_p \sum_k (d_i - y_i - J_i\delta)^2$$

Next the error term can be written as:

$$E(W + \delta) \cong \left\| \bar{y} - \bar{d} - J\delta \right\|^2 \tag{76}$$

To minimize this function, one takes the derivative and sets it to zero. The derivative of the above function set to zero becomes:

$-2J^T(\bar{d} - \bar{y} - J\delta) = 0$, namely:

$J^T(\bar{y} - \bar{d}) = J^T J\delta$

The rate of change can be tempered by a scalar multiple shown by parameter η. Equation (76) can be written as:

$J^T(\bar{y} - \bar{d}) = (J^T J + \eta I)\delta$, or as:

$J^T E = (J^T J + \eta I)\delta$

where I is the identity matrix. It can be seen that the rate of change in weights can be computed by:

$\delta = \dfrac{J^T E}{(J^T J + \eta I)}$

It can be easily seen that the weights for the next iteration can be computed using the following equation:

$$W_{t+1} = W_t - (J_t^T J_t + \eta_t I)^{-1} J_t^T E_t \tag{77}$$

Where J is the Jacobian (a matrix of first order derivatives) of m input errors with respect to n weights of the neural network, I is the identity matrix and η_t is the learning parameter.

Chapter 9

Using Committee of Models to Improve Analytical Accuracy

The traditional data-driven prediction methods have constructed multiple models and selected the one with the best performance, discarding all the others. This approach has some disadvantages: 1) the effort of constructing several models is wasted, 2) the selected model may not consistently perform most accurately or be robust on all types of data and with diverse types of disease predictions, 3) the selected algorithm may not be able to sustain or perform consistently on training data types as changes to data types occur over time. To overcome these disadvantages, this book proposes a multi-model ensemble (also known as committee of models) approach which combines multiple algorithms with a weighted sum formulation. This framework considered five different ensemble schemes and compared their performance on the DVT case study data set. These schemes include a voting formula, two accuracy-based weighting schemes, a diversity-based weighting and optimization-based weighting. The goal of constructing ensembles is to identify the weights of each algorithm such that it improves data-driven prognostics performance.

The case study employed in this book demonstrates that the ensemble approach provides a more accurate prediction than a single algorithm. Given a number of neural networks to select from, the goal is to select a weighted sum of these models' output that provides the most accurate classification. An oracle program can be defined to select the most accurate algorithm from a set of five ensembles (or committee) of algorithms provided by the four ANN models. An oracle is defined as an overseer which selects the most appropriate answer amongst a set of options. An oracle, is a program that selects a prediction from among a number of ensembles or models that meet a desired level of accuracy or predictive characteristic of a disease.

Since one model performs better in predicting true positives and another better at predicting the true negatives, this book proposes the oracle program to combine the predictions from models in a way that the model with higher accuracy is assigned a higher weight and the worst model still contributes to the prediction but at a smaller weight. This way, the oracle can improve the classification accuracy, sensitivity and specificity by combining the best classification characteristics from different models.

Given that there are many neural networks to select from, the goal is to select the most accurate model, or ensemble of models for prediction of a particular disease. Let's as an example suppose that the prognostics engine trains four different algorithms to make a prediction for DVT. It can then build five different ensembles with different weighted sum from the four models' output. The prognostics engine trains another four models to predict a different disease and builds another set of five ensembles. For each disease, a different set of ensembles are constructed. Then the prognostics engine uses an oracle, an overseer program that selects the most accurate ensemble for each disease prediction.

In prior research, a meta-classifier is used to compose a prediction from the four models based on a linear combination of the characteristics that are desired in the final classification. A meta-classifier is a computational tool that integrates in some principled fashion the separately trained classifiers to boost overall predictive accuracy (Prodormidis, Chan, Stolfo 2000). In this framework, this meta-classifier is called the oracle program. The oracle program can be set up to enhance any of the four desired accuracy characteristics: either directly improve True Positives (TP), True Negatives (TN), False Positives (FP) or False Negatives (FN), or to improve other accuracy measurements such as sensitivity, specificity or Youden's *J* index.

In this framework, a positive case is a patient with illness and a TP classification means the algorithm has correctly classified the ill patient as sick. Then FP represents Type I error (α) and FN represents Type II error (β) as shown in Figure 9.1.

		Truth	
		Sick	Healthy
Test	Sick	TP (1- β)	FP α
	Healthy	FN β	TN (1- α)

Fig. 9.1 - Truth Table indicating Type I and Type II errors

It's important to define the objectives for the oracle program. The practitioner must define the selection criteria for the oracle program; is the oracle to select a model or ensemble of models that reduce Type I (FP) error, or Type II (FN) error, or both errors; or as it will be presented later, a combination of accuracy measures.

While in most situations, the criteria calls for lower Type II error, in certain situations where the population is large and the cost of treatment is high, the criteria would include reducing Type I error as well.

The oracle program can be set up to provide a meta-classification based on a linear combination of these characteristics. The goal of the ensemble is to produce a synthesized classification result based on weighted sum of ANN models as:

$$\hat{p} = \sum_{j=1}^{K}(w_j p_j) \tag{78}$$

The assumption in this book is that the ensemble consists of K models, and p_j is the prediction of model j. The result of the ensemble's prediction is represented by $\hat{p}$.

9.1 Vote-based Schema

Voting approach selects the final results based on majority vote on a specific accuracy dimension or result category. For example, if the goal is to minimize FN, then one must consider a voting schema that produces the lowest FN among the four models on a given new case data set. The voting schema works as follows: Run all four models on the new data set. Select the lowest FN count, or select a weight sum of models that produce the lowest FN+FP count.

A hybrid schema can work by defining a relative preference ratio. The assumption is that models with more correct prediction are preferred over the other models. The relative preference of a model is determined by the number of correct predictions minus incorrect predictions. This schema was used for Ensemble #1. The mathematical representation of schema for Ensemble#1 is shown in (79) and (80). This ensemble assumes n data cases and K models in the ensemble:

$$model\ j\ score = \sum_{i=1}^{n}(correct\ predictions - incorrect\ predictions) \tag{79}$$

$$w_j = \frac{model\ j\ score}{\sum_{i=1}^{K} model\ i\ score} \tag{80}$$

As shown in this equation, the intent is to find the weights according to the ratio of preference for a model that provides higher accuracy (lower FN count).

9.2 Accuracy-based Ensemble Schema

Accuracy-based ensemble seeks to find a weighted sum of algorithms that minimize error. For example, if the intent is to find the lowest FN, one can define the error for each validation case as follows. Let's assume that T_i is the truth of a particular validation case, and p_{ij} is the prediction rendered by algorithm j for case i. Also assume that there are a total of K different algorithms. Ensemble #2, attempts to increase the number of TP count by defining the number of errors for each model j:

Then one can define the total error count by:

$$\varepsilon_j = \sum_{i=1}^{n} \varepsilon(p_{ij}, T_i) \tag{81}$$

where $\varepsilon(p_{ij}, T_i)$ equals to 1 if p_{ij} does not match the truth T_i, or equals to zero if prediction matches the truth.

Then one can define the weight of algorithm j for ensemble #1 with the goal of increasing the quantity of TP. Assuming that the total number of TP from a model j is shown by TP_j, it's possible to define the weights by:

$$w_j = \frac{(TP_j)}{\sum_{j=1}^{m}(TP_j)} \tag{82}$$

For ensemble#3, one can define the weight of algorithm j with the goal of reducing the quantity of FN error:

$$w_j = \frac{(\varepsilon_j)^{-1}}{\sum_{j=1}^{K}(\varepsilon_j)^{-1}} \tag{83}$$

In this framework, two ensembles, Ensemble#2 and Ensemble#3 used accuracy-based scheme to determine the weights. The results are discussed and compared in Chapter 5.

9.3 Diversity-based Schema

The accuracy-based weighted sum formulation exclusively relies on accuracy to compute the weights. However, one can argue that accuracy is not the only factor that affects ensemble performance. The diversity-based schema measures the extent to which the predictions by one model are distinguishable from predictions by other models. The diversity-based schema increases the robustness performance of the ensemble. Said differently, this ensemble assigns higher weight to the model with higher prediction diversity because it offers higher ensemble robustness. Let's assume that n data sets are employed to train and validate all k models. One can compute a prediction error term u_j to correspond to uniqueness of the model j:

$$\theta_j = (p_{j1} - T_1, \dots, p_{jn} - T_n) \tag{84}$$

Given k algorithms, it's possible to define the error vector of $\theta_1, \theta_2, \dots, \theta_K$. The diversity of the jth model can be computed as the sum of Euclidean distances between the vector θ_j and all other error vectors, defined by:

$$D_j = \sum_{i=1; j \neq i}^{K} \|\theta_j - \theta_i\| \tag{85}$$

The prediction diversity determines how a model's result is distinguishable from those of other models. Let's compute a normalized weight w_j for the jth model in the ensemble by:

$$w_j = \frac{D_j}{\sum_{i=1}^{k} D_i} \tag{86}$$

Ensemble#4 uses diversity-based schema.

9.4 Optimization-based Schema

One proposal in this book is to define the oracle (meta-classifier) as an optimization model. The optimization-based schema can take into account both the accuracy-based as well as the diversity-based weighting scheme to improve accuracy and robustness. This method is adapted from Hu, et al. (Hu, Youn, Wang 2010). In optimization-based schema one can write Eq. (78) as:

$$minimize\ \varepsilon\left(\sum_{j=1}^{K}(w_j\, p_{ij}), T_i\right) \tag{87}$$

$$\sum_{j=1}^{K} w_j = 1., \quad \text{and} \quad w_j \geq 0 \ for\ all\ j = 1, \dots K \tag{88}$$

Where w_j is the weight of model p_j and T_i is the expected result for the ith data set. The objective function attempts to minimize the difference between the expected result and the weighted sum of each model's result. Ensemble#5 uses optimization-based schema. The weights w_1, w_2, w_3 and w_4 corresponding to each of the four analytical models were determined using the optimization model in Excel Solver as is illustrated in Figure 40.

PART III:

Case Study

Chapter 10

Data Types, Data Requirements and Data Pre-Processing

Researchers have studied machine learning, classification and training adaptive methods to data, and have identified two approaches to learning: programmed and concept attainment. Programmed learning is applicable when the researcher knows the underlying causal relationships in the system and the data. The concept attainment is an adaptive learning approach where a system learns from *a priori* set of examples and thus retains concepts from prior data sets, in other words it learns by classifying patterns in the input data. This framework applies the concept attainment type of learning using ANNs as the learning models. A concept can be described as a mapping between an input data set and a clinical outcome.

Some interesting research questions arise that merit a full investigation elsewhere, but are discussed briefly here:

A) How much data is adequate for learning to predict a given disease?
B) How much of the error in prediction can be attributed to noise in data versus the model that captures the concept or due to the change in concept?
C) What pre-processing methods are applied to measured data to prepare data for learning algorithms?

The answers are briefly discussed as follows:

10.1 How much data is adequate for learning to predict a given disease?

In order to train a Prognostics engine adequately, the ideal data set must consist of adequate number of both positive and negative cases of disease (Principe, Euliano, Lefebvre 1999). From experience, some basic rules of thumb have been developed for determining the amount of data needed for proper training of ANN models. The rules have been developed as guidelines by ANN experts (Principe 2011).

1. A data set must have a minimum of 5 times as many exemplars (data sets) as the number of weights in the ANN model. For example, in the DVT model that includes 20 input variables, and 4 layers of network, there can be as many as 60 weights. Thus the minimum number of input data should be somewhere around 300 rows of data.

2. The data set must have approximately 50 times the number of exemplars (data sets) than features. A feature is the number of columns. In the DVT model that includes 20 columns, it's recommended to need a minimum of 1000 rows of data (50 times more rows than columns)

3. In classification models, the number of rows in the smallest class should be preferably 5 times the number of input columns. For example, in the DVT model that has two classifications (disease or no-disease), the number of data rows in the smaller class must be over 100 rows.

In order to properly train a model, it's recommended to include equal number of positive and negative cases to have a balanced network. Let's suppose the goal is to train a model with 400 negative cases and only 50 positive cases, the ANN model naturally works to minimize errors. As a result, the model gets trained by the input data such that minimizing errors for the 400 cases overshadows the minimizing errors for the 50 positive cases. So, it's recommended to randomly select 50 cases from negative and 50 cases from negative sample and train on this set.

How much of the error in prediction can be attributed to noise in data versus the model that captures the concept or due to the change in concept?

Data noise can be caused by incorrect measurements of patient physiological data, disruptions to measurements (missing data) and or incorrect *a priori* classification or units of measure. Concept changes on the other hand can be attributed to changes to how patients, medications and treatment protocols and practices change over time. For example, certain diseases develop resistance to certain drugs over time so those drugs are not as effective, or the procedures for a treatment change that make it either more or less effective, but it's prescribed by same name.

By conducting a comparison of results of four different ANN models, the difference in accuracy among the models can give us some clues to the amount of error that can be attributed to the model.

What pre-processing tools are used to prepare measured data for learning algorithms?

In most neural network models, all data in each column is normalized such that an amplitude and an offset is applied to the data of each column. It's important to study the data before training a model. If the input data ranges are vastly different (for example, one data column has a range of 1000 and another has a range of 1), then the errors from multiplying weights by inputs that have a large range will overtake the smaller data range.

10.2 Input Data Pre-Processing

The goal of pre-processing is to bring the range of input data values within a computationally acceptable range for the ANN computations. ANNS train faster and perform better if their data is pre-processed. The same pre-processing must be applied to test data. Data scaling is an important pre-processing step before training ANNs. Data scaling equalizes the importance of input variables at the input layer. For example, if one input variables ranges between 1 and 10,000 and another ranges between 0.001 and 0.1, the network should be able to use proper initial weights, namely small weights for the first variable but larger weights for the second variable. But, data scaling make the choice of initial weights for ANNs easier so they can train faster.

At the input layer, several methods are available to pre-process the measured data for ANN models. These methods include:

1. **Moving average:** Computes the moving average of a column using the chosen window length.
2. **Difference:** Computes the difference or percent difference along a column of data from the mean of the column.
3. **Clip data:** Clip data to a given max value or min value
4. **Log of data:** Takes logarithm of each data item
5. **Mean and Variance:** Normalize the data by fixing the mean to zero and use variance of from the mean to scale the data

A commonly used scaling method normalizes input data to unit length. Normalizing to unit length implies that the sum of squares of values in a given data set must equal to 1. To normalize each data value, the following steps are taken:

1. Square all data values in a given data set

2. Sum the squares. Take square root of the sum of squares
3. Divide each data item in the data set by this square root of sum of squares. The result of each division is a normalized data item.

Other pre-processing and coding techniques are necessary for categorical data. For example, let's assume a particular patient data is recorded as a categorical input variable such that it takes values of Very Low, Low, Medium, High and Very High. This variable should not be coded in numeric values of 0.0, 0.25, 0.50, 0.75, 1.00, as this would create incorrect interpretations by the ANN model. For example, it would incorrectly imply that a High category is exactly 3 times more than a Low value. Such input variables are coded and transformed into binary inputs. In this example, the categorical values would be mapped as shown in Table 10.1:

Table 10.1. Coding example of categorical data

Category	Binary Input
Very Low	0 0 0 0
Low	1 0 0 0
Medium	1 1 0 0
High	1 1 1 0
Very High	1 1 1 1

Additional data pre-processing occur at each layer of ANN models. After each layer, the range of normalized values is determined by the range of outputs of the nonlinear transfer functions (activation function) used by the model. For example, if a *Tanh* axon is used, the data output is normalized to a range between -1 and +1. If the data for the column is already in the desired range, then the amplitude will be 1 and the offset will be 0, so that the normalized data will be the same as the original data. There are other options that clean and randomize data depending on what is intended for the initial data processing. Some example methods are:

- **Randomize rows:** Randomly re-arrange rows of data.
- **Clean data:** replace missing or corrupted data with an average of the column, ore the most recurring data or the nearest value in the column.

The measured data may come from a number of acquisition devices and data bases. Each training set is represented by input data vector **X** and a prognostic disease **Z**, so one can represent each training set as $\{(x_1, z_1), ..., (x_n, z_n)\}$ for some unknown function **Z = P(X)**. Each x_i is a set of attributes (feature) vector **X** of the form $\{x_{i1}, x_{i2}, ..., x_{ik}\}$, and each z_i represents the prognostic disease label associated with each vector ($Z_i \in \{z_1, z_2, ..., z_n\}$). Our task is to compute a classifier or model $\hat{P}$ that approximates **P** and correctly labels any feature vector drawn from the same vector source as the training set.

Once the data is collected into a single data base, called Memory, it can be used to train several classifiers that can classify a new data set into a number of disease types. This framework trained four classifier models using N-leave-out method. In this approach, each model is trained on a portion of the data and leave *N* data sets out of training to be used for testing. This process continues until all data sets have been used training and testing. This training approach reduces the effect of data bias.

10.3 Data Acquisition for ANN models

ANN models require real time data acquisition from several sources including patient vital sign monitors, lab results, waveform data, data acquired from clinical instruments, genetic sequence data, medical record and other diagnostic tests. The challenge with managing a diverse set of data can be described in the taxonomy shown in Table 10.2. As explained in this table, analysis must consider all types of data in real time as each data source is updated. In this framework 1,073 cases were analyzed with are adequate for proper training of ANN models.

Table 10.2. Clinical Data Types Are Diverse

Nominal	Ordinal	Ratio	Fuzzy - Range	Image	Signal	Graph	Clinical Charts
Male	High	34.22					
Female	Low	?					
. . .	. . .	. . .	. . .	. . .	. . .	. . .	. . .
Male	High	-5.70					

The input file for each ANN model must accommodate the necessary medical data types from the taxonomy above. The challenge is handling images, missing data elements (when there is interruption to measuring clinical information) and various types of clinical charts. The goal is to extract the relevant medical data from images and charts in form of discrete data elements. Signal and Range data can be represented by time-series data and data matrix format.

10.4 Case Study: Application of ANN to DVT/PE Data

Patients in acute care can develop a multitude of complications ranging from pulmonary, respiratory and digestive to infections. The goal of this framework is to collect such data in 1 minute intervals and study the changes in data to predict patient's health condition using ANN models developed for each type of complication. The challenge is to run the models in real time, once every minute as new data becomes available. The choice of time window can vary from several minutes to several hours. The ANN models dedicated to each human physiological system predict complications in each category. The physicians can apply the appropriate treatment before such complications occur or escalate. Similarly, this book explores the application of such ANN models to signal early indications as to whether treatments are being effective.

The precursor to Pulmonary Embolism is thrombosis, formation of blood clots inside a blood vessel obstructing the flow of blood. There are three causal elements that lead to blood clot disposition. These are known as the Virchow's triad (Virchow 1856):

- Abnormal blood flow. Abnormal blood flow is affected by narrowing of the vessels. Narrowing of the blood vessels causes turbulence that lead to formation of blood clots.

- Injuries to the vascular endothelium. Injuries to the vascular interior wall can be caused by damage to the veins arising from surgery or hypertension.
- Abnormal constitution of blood. The constituents of blood, such as proteins, water components and other elements are out of balance increasing blood thickness and propensity to form clots.

A rubric for calculating patient's risk of developing Pulmonary Embolism (PE) is known as Wells score (Wells, Anderson, et al. 1997). Wells score provides the probability that a patient might develop pulmonary embolism. It uses the following criteria:

- Are there clinical signs and symptoms of DVT?
- Is pulmonary embolism the top diagnosis?
- Is heart rate over 100?
- Is patient immobilized at least 3 days?
- Was a surgical procedure done in the last 4 weeks?
- Was patient previously diagnosed with PE or DVT?
- Is patient Hemoptysis (coughs-up blood)?
- Does patient have malignancy with treatment within 6 months or is palliative?

The goal of predicting DVT is to use data, measurements of the pre-cursors or risk factors to provide predictions about blood clot formations. The research hypothesis is that one can predict DVT in advance using data about patient's clinical data.

Finally, Deep Vein Thrombosis (DVT) is a condition that often occurs with patients with long periods of rest in hospitals. A DVT is a blood clot that forms in a vein deep in the body, often in the lower leg or thigh. A blood clot in a deep vein can break off and travel through the blood stream. The loose blood clot is called embolus. When the clot reaches the lungs and blocks blood flow, the condition is called pulmonary embolism (PE).

When PE is severe it causes lungs to collapse and leads to heart failure. One in every hundred people who develop DVT dies. According to some estimates, more than 900,000 Americans develop DVT each year and 500,000 of them develop PE with 30% of those cases being fatal. About two-thirds of all DVT events are related to hospitalization. The National Quality Forum (NQF) in its 2006 update reports that DVT is the third most common cause of hospital-related deaths in the US and the most common preventable cause of hospital death.

The data collected in this case study is typically gathered over several days. The data set includes a wide range of qualitative and quantitative clinical test results and reports.

One aim of this framework was to determine viability of ANN models to predict patients' susceptibility to acquire DVT/PE.

According to StopDVT.org (2011), the risk factors for DVT/PE are the following:

- Age: over 40 years
- Already had blood clots
- Family history of blood clots
- Suffering from or had treatment for cancer
- Certain blood diseases

- Being treated for heart failure and circulation problems
- Experienced recent surgery in particular in the hips or knees
- Have inherited clotting tendency
- Who are very tall

DVT is also common among women who are:

- Pregnant
- Recently had a baby
- Taking contraceptive pill
- On hormone replacement therapy (HRT)

The progress of acquiring DVT/PE is shown in Figure 10.1. The important factors include the type of surgery, length of surgery, whether the patient was put on chemical prophylaxis and whether mechanical (SCD) devices were employed and how well the chemical prophylaxis were administered during the patient stay.

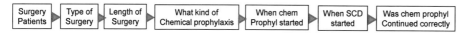

Fig. 10.1 - Progression of patient health status who present with DVT/PE

The initial study considered a sample of over a thousand patients of which 225 (approximately 21%) had developed DVT/PE. Three different off-the-shelf artificial neural network tools for this study were evaluated using this data set. To perform algorithm training, a software package was used that offered supervised learning, ability to perform K-fold cross validation, and extensive post-test accuracy and cross-validation results after each training session.

The input data consisted of 24 different dimensions based on patient demographic and clinical elements such as: AGE, WEIGHT, GENDER, Encounter type (Outpatient, Inpatient), length of stay, Stay over 48HOURS (TRUE or FALSE), ICU vs. Acute Care patient, BMI (BioMass Index) Level, Blood measures (Platelets count, RBC, Hematocrit, Hemoglobin), other blood related values obtained from lab test results, International Normalized Ratio, an indicator of coagulation (INR of 2-3 is preferred but varies by patient), Glucose levels, and related test results, and DVT/PE Result (1 for positive, 0 for negative). For the specific case study, a sample data from patient electronic medical record systems was collected, and then completely anonymized so there was no identifiable information.

To build an ANN model, a typical neural tool undergoes 4 stages for data analysis and training:

1. Data set Manager. In this stage the scope of data fields for the model are set

2. Train. The model is trained to identify its internal neural network weights

3. Test. This stage determines how robust the model is given the set of data

4. Predict. In this stage, the trained model is applied to a new patient data set for prediction.

Once the model was trained on historical patient data, the trained model was applied to a new set of data for new patients during their stay in the hospital. The model has the ability to predict each patient's propensity to develop DVT/PE. The predictions are denoted by a '1' to denote patient is at risk of developing DVT/PE or '0' indicating that the DVT/PE risks are very low for the patient. When the prediction indicates risks of developing DVT/PE, then certain interventions such as medications and physical means are prescribed by the physician to the patient.

ANN models are known for their resilience to missing data. The model can fill-in the fields with missing data items. The same model can be setup to run periodically every few minutes (or every hour) for several days on the same patient but on new datasets as they're generated from the electronic medical record.

Furthermore, the model provides the input weights that it applies to compute predictions. Knowing the weights is helpful in several ways:

1. It can point to the importance of certain input variables over other variables and improves our understanding of which factors contribute to DVT/PE the most, and

2. Aid in developing hypotheses for further studies that enhance evidence-based medicine, in particular studies that determine which intervention methods have been most successful in preventing DVT/PE.

In the training of the neural net three factors were considered: error calculation, topology selection and prevent over-training. Error measures were computed as Mean Squared Error over all the training cases, in other words the mean squared difference between the correct answer and the answer given by the net. Through classification, the result is more than one output for each training case (one output corresponding to each dependent category). The tool allows computing the Mean Squared Error over all the outputs for all the training cases in comparison to the desired output values.

The topology is determined based on the best net configuration that produces the best training result. A typical network consists of a single hidden layer. The model automatically adds a number of neurons in each layer and additional layers to determine which topology learns the relationship between the independent variables and the dependent variable (response) the best (by having the lowest error). By default the model uses 2- to 6 hidden layers. Larger models could take several hours to train. But, once the model is trained, predictions can be computed in a few seconds. Most models can be trained in two hidden layers.

Overtraining occurs when the number of iterations increases beyond the initial training such that the model's synaptic weights and topology match the problem specifically and the model is no longer generalizable to other datasets, namely the model does not apply to cases not included in the training. One approach to avoid "over-training" is the test-while-training method. In this approach the model is tested immediately after every iteration of training then the error gets measured. If the error starts to grow, it's indication that the researcher is starting to over-train the model.

The detailed description of input data types are presented in Table 10.3. As shown in the table, each data field is either independent numeric or independent category, except for one data type that represent the dependent variable. The goal of the model is to predict the dependent variable (DVT/PE Result). The third column indicates which input variables were selected by the initial training models as significant variables. These significant variables were used as input variable to train the final four models.

There are four steps for building and running an ANN model.

• Step1: Define and manage the input layer data. Define the data types, independent variables and the dependent variable.

- Step 2: Train the model on a sample of cases (typically 100 cases are sufficient for training, but more cases will help reduce percent of bad predictions)
- Step 3: Test the model using the same set of training cases plus additional cases.
- Step 4: Run the model. Observe the error rate and percent of bad predictions.

Table 10.3 - Input Data fields and their type

Data Variable	Variable Type	Significant to ANN Training
CASE_ID	Not Used	
CREATED_DT	Not Used	
VISIT DATE	Not Used	
AGE	Independent Numeric	Yes
Length of Stay (days)	Independent Numeric	Yes
Weight (Kg)	Independent Numeric	Yes
BMI Index	Independent Numeric	Yes
IS INPATIENT?	Independent Category	
Is Adult?	Independent Category	
Maximum Glucose	Independent Numeric	
Minimum Glucose	Independent Numeric	
Maximum Platelets	Independent Numeric	
Minimum Platelets	Independent Numeric	Yes
Maximum INR	Independent Numeric	Yes
Minimum INR	Independent Numeric	Yes
Maximum RBC	Independent Numeric	
Minimum RBC	Independent Numeric	
Maximum Hb	Independent Numeric	Yes
Minimum Hb	Independent Numeric	
Maximum HCT	Independent Numeric	Yes
Minimum HCT	Independent Numeric	
Maximum MCH	Independent Numeric	
Minimum MCH	Independent Numeric	
Maximum MCHC	Independent Numeric	
Minimum MCHC	Independent Numeric	
Maximum RDW-CV1	Independent Numeric	
Maximum RDW-CV2	Independent Numeric	Yes
Minimum Diastolic BP	Independent Numeric	Yes
Maximum Diastolic BP	Independent Numeric	
Maximum Systolic BP	Independent Numeric	
Minimum Systolic BP	Independent Numeric	
Smoker?	Independent Category	Yes

DVT/PE RESULT	Dependent Numeric	

A typical output screen of model training, cross validation and testing along with results are presented in Figure 10.2 as example. Note the mix of numeric and categorical independent variables. The dependent variable is the DVT/PE Result column. There were 1,073 independent patient cases in the data set, of which there were 225 confirmed positive cases of DVT. The algorithm trained on 1,073 cases. The data for the purpose of this case study were simulated. Then it was tested for accuracy on an N-Leave-Out method, using 2% of data cases in each iteration for cross validation. The results of one model are shown in Figure 10.2 only as illustration of typical output. A typical output of cross validation shows a confusion matrix, ROC curve and other calculations including sensitivity and specificity for a range of thresholds.

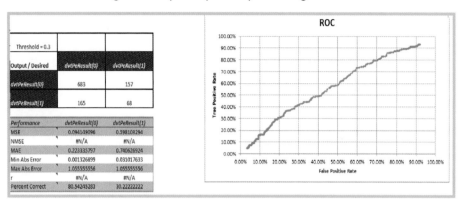

Threshold = 0.3		
Output / Desired	dvtPeResult(0)	dvtPeResult(1)
dvtPeResult(0)	683	157
dvtPeResult(1)	165	68

Performance	dvtPeResult(0)	dvtPeResult(1)
MSE	0.094149096	0.598103294
NMSE	#N/A	#N/A
MAE	0.223335797	0.740626924
Min Abs Error	0.001326899	0.031017633
Max Abs Error	1.055555556	1.055555556
r	#N/A	#N/A
Percent Correct	80.54245283	30.22222222

ROC Detection Threshold	Total Detections	True Positive (TP)	False Positive (FP)	True Negative (TN)	False Negative (FN)	Detected as Positive ((TP+FP)/(TP+FP+TN+FN))	False Positive Rate (FP/(FP+TN))	True Positive Rate (TP/(TP+FN))	False Discovery Rate (FP/(FP+TP))
0.001	991	210	781	67	15	92.36%	92.10%	93.33%	78.81%
0.002	991	210	781	67	15	92.36%	92.10%	93.33%	78.81%
0.003	989	210	779	69	15	92.17%	91.86%	93.33%	78.77%
0.004	988	210	778	70	15	92.08%	91.75%	93.33%	78.74%
0.005	985	210	775	73	15	91.80%	91.39%	93.33%	78.68%
0.006	985	210	775	73	15	91.80%	91.39%	93.33%	78.68%
0.007	985	210	775	73	15	91.80%	91.39%	93.33%	78.68%
0.008	985	210	775	73	15	91.80%	91.39%	93.33%	78.68%
0.009	984	209	775	73	16	91.71%	91.39%	92.89%	78.76%
0.01	984	209	775	73	16	91.71%	91.39%	92.89%	78.76%
0.011	984	209	775	73	16	91.71%	91.39%	92.89%	78.76%
0.012	983	209	774	74	16	91.61%	91.27%	92.89%	78.74%
0.013	983	209	774	74	16	91.61%	91.27%	92.89%	78.74%
0.014	983	209	774	74	16	91.61%	91.27%	92.89%	78.74%
0.015	982	209	773	75	16	91.52%	91.16%	92.89%	78.72%
0.016	980	209	771	77	16	91.33%	90.92%	92.89%	78.67%
0.017	979	208	771	77	17	91.24%	90.92%	92.44%	78.75%

Fig. 10.2 - Output screen from NeuroSolutions after training on 1,073 patient cases

Four different algorithms were used to train four independent models on the same data set. The data was randomized by the ANN tool in the first step. In the second step, a Greedy Search ANN algorithm was used to identify the significant input variables. The number of input variables was reduced from 29 to 12 according to the selection made by the first stage ANN model.

In the case of multi-layer perceptron (MLP) algorithm, the search for the optimum training led to finding the optimum number of layers. The tool was configured to find the optimum number of layers as it constructed several multi-layer networks and compared the Mean Square Error of the MLP networks. The model configurations consisted of 2-node, 3-node, 4-node, 5-node and 6-node arrangements. The tool selected the optimum number of layers that provided the lowest MSE. The largest number of iterations occurred with the 6-node model with 150 iterations. The model completed training and running in 40minutes on a dual core Intel processor desktop computer (2.8GHz CPU speed).

Training each model required separate training, cross-validation and testing process. The models consumed several "epochs" to complete the training. An epoch is representation of an entire training set in neural networks, namely the number of iterations of training required for the model to reach its global optimum solution. The model training stops when the change in Mean Square Error (MSE) reaches a small threshold defined by the user. Table 10.4 shows the number of epochs that each model took for training. This table compares the relative efficiency of each neural network model.

Table 10.4. Computational Resources consumed by each model

Model	Epochs
MLP- LM	20
GFN-LM	20
SVM	150
PNN	3

A sensitivity analysis was performed to determine the significance of input variables. This testing process provides a measure of the relative importance among the inputs of the neural model and illustrates how the model output varies in response to variation of an input. Sensitivity analysis works by taking an input and varying it between its mean, ± a (user-defined) number of standard deviations while all other inputs are fixed at their respective means. The network output is computed for a user-defined number of steps above and below the mean. This process is repeated for each input and the impact on output is recorded at each step. An alternate variation of this process is to vary the input of interest between its minimum value and its maximum value. This option is especially useful for binary inputs or inputs which have a non-Gaussian distribution.

The result of sensitivity analysis is shown in Figure 10.3. This figure shows the relative strength of weights of input variables. Of these variables, Minimum and Maximum INR, followed by patient Weight, Length of stay, Maximum RDW-CV2, Patient age were most significant input variables toward classification of patients.

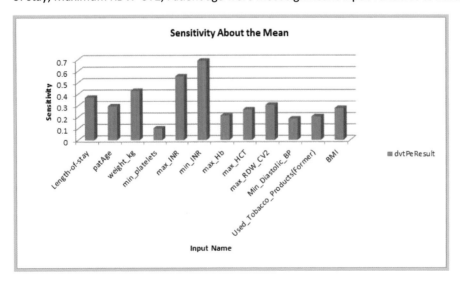

196

Fig. 10.3 - Strength of Input variables towards classification

The results point to several variables as being significant in predicting DVT/PE. The sensitivity analysis provided the following ranking of the input variables based on their significance towards patient classification:

1. Minimum INR
2. Maximum INR
3. Weight
4. Length of Stay
5. Maximum RDW-CV2
6. Patient Age

Sensitivity analysis performed using the software package reveals the degree that one variable impacts the output. It does not determine if the changes in input are positively or negatively correlated. A clinical interpretation of the sensitivity analysis can be given as follows: The INR values explain the patient's blood characteristics. It makes sense that sensitivity analysis has pinpointed Minimum and Maximum INR as significant inputs to classification. INR, a standard measure of blood clotting characteristics indicates the blood tendency to form clots. A lower INR correlates with higher chance of blood clot formation. The significance of RDW-CV2 can be explained as it's a property of red blood cells that correspond to the width of red blood cells. Wider blood cells are more likely to be caught in capillaries, blocking blood flow. Length of Stay is significant as it's empirically observed that longer patient's stay in hospital is correlated with increase in frequency of DVT, but only for a certain length of stay. The relationship between Length of Stay and occurrence of DVT follows a quadratic equation. Patient Weight might point to certain underlying patient characteristics which could related to the patient's lower levels of mobility or other factors yet unknown. Of these variables, the blood related measurements point to possible opportunities for clinical intervention through medication.

But, the benefit of sensitivity analysis is that it highlights those significant variables which can be further studied in future research to determine causal relevance to a particular disease. Unlike prior research such as Well's CPR method that choose input variables in somewhat arbitrary method, neural network models constructed in this framework can reveal a data-driven approach through sensitivity analysis to identify the significant input variables among a large list of input variables.

Chapter 11

Analytics Accuracy

In order to present a meaningful and practical overview of accuracy, I'll over a real clinical prediction case study as the backdrop. Consider a clinical case study consisting over a 1,000 patient cases. Of this population of patients who were admitted to a hospital for various treatments of which 225 had developed positive cases of DVT. The patient data consisted of 29 independent variables and one dependent variable. The input data included various relevant physical and vital sign data ranging from blood pressure to heart rate and blood lab test results. The input variables consisted of both continuous and dichotomous variables. The dependent variable was a dichotomous variable that represented the clinical outcome, the occurrence or absence of a disease. In this study, the output was defined by a marker called Deep Vein Thrombosis (DVT).

DVT is the formation of blood clots in deep veins, typically in leg veins. Blood clots can dislodge and flow to lungs causing a more critical condition called Pulmonary Embolism (PE). DVT/PE is a serious medical condition that can cause serious pain and even death. In the US alone approximately 350,000 to 600,000 patients suffer from DVT and at least 100,000 deaths per year are attributed to DVT/PE (The Surgeon General's Call to Action to Prevent Deep Vein Thrombosis and Pulmonary Embolism, 2008).

Neural networks have been successfully applied to classify patterns based on learning from prior examples. Different neural network models use different learning rules, but in general they determine pattern statistics from a set of training examples and then classify new data according to the trained rules. Stated differently, a trained neural network model classifies (or maps) a set of input data to a specific disease from a set of diseases.

Four models were trained and tested in two stages: in the first stage, a genetic, greedy search neural network algorithm was employed to identify the input variables with most predictive power. It narrowed the list of input variables from 29 down to 12 variables. In the second stage, all four models were trained and tested on the 12 input variables that were selected by the genetic algorithm model (obtained from stage 1). The list of the most significant predictive variables was provided in Table 7. Next in Table 11.1, a description of significant input variables is provided.

Table 11.1 - Input variables description

Input Variable	Data Type	Definition
AGE	Continuous	Patient's age
INPATIENT	Dichotomous	Is patient admitted as inpatient?
WEIGHT	Continuous	Weight during stay in Kg.
MIN PLATELET	Continuous	Minimum no. of blood platelets, tiny cells that assist in blood clotting
MIN INR	Continuous	Minimum INR (International Normalized Ratio). The standard for a healthy person is 1.
MAX INR	Continuous	Maximum INR (International Normalized Ratio).
MAX Hemoglobin	Continuous	Maximum Hemoglobin concentration. The average for humans is 16 g/100ml.
MIN DIASTOLIC BP	Continuous	Minimum blood pressure when heart is at rest. A normal diastolic BP is under 80, but over 90 is considered hypertension.
MAX HCT	Continuous	Maximum hematocrit: the proportion, by volume, of

		red blood cells
MAX RDW CV2	Continuous	Minimum red blood cell distribution width.
BMI Index	Continuous	BioMass Index, a measure of weight and height, values between 18.5-24.9 are regarded normal weight
SMOKER	Categorical	Patient's smoking status as either Former, Unknown, or Current Smoker

11.1 Computational Method

In this framework, four different prediction and classification algorithms were trained and tested on 12 data input variables and 1,073 patient cases. The data for the purpose of this case study were simulated. There were 89 true positive cases in the retrospective study. For each of the four models, the "Leave-N-out" technique was employed. This technique is a combined training and cross-validation method used to minimize bias due to random data selection. This approach trains the network multiple times, each time omitting a different subset of the data and using that subset for validation. The outputs from each tested subset are combined into one testing report and the model is trained one final time using all of the data.

The test results of all four models can be compared using classification measures such as number of false positives (FP), false negatives (FN), true positives (TP) and true negatives (TN). The performance of four ANN models is shown in Table 11.2.

Table11.2 - Model test results

Model	TP	FP	TN	FN	Total
Probabilistic Neural Network	94	216	632	131	1,073
Support Vector Machines	98	230	618	127	1,073
Multi-layer Perceptron with LM	90	213	635	135	1,073
Generalized Feed forward with LM	129	336	512	96	1,073

11.2 Accuracy and Validation

External validity of medical prediction models is an extremely challenging task. Clinical validation is challenging not just because it involves prospective patient studies, double-blind studies and careful administration of research protocols, but for two other reasons: first, if the model predicts a disease and the patient gets the treatment per recommendation of the predictive model, we can't determine if the patient would have exhibited the predicted disease to confirm our prediction. In other words, the medical treatment masks the possible outcome. Second and in contrary, if the model predicts no disease but the patient gets treatment, we would not be able to invalidate the model's prediction since we can't claim that the disease might have occurred.

This framework focuses on internal validity in terms of accuracy but leaves external (clinical) validation to future research projects. Several measurements have been proposed as methods for internal validation. Some of the measurements that are commonly used to compare accuracy of classification models include:

Accuracy, Sensitivity, Specificity, Area Under Receiver Operating Curve (AUROC) and Likelihood Ratio (LR). *Sensitivity* measures the fraction of positive cases that are classified correctly as positive.

Specificity is the fraction of negative cases that are classified correctly as negative. AUROC is the area under the ROC and is regarded as a good overall measure of predictive accuracy of a model (Bewick, Cheek, Ball 2004). An ROC can be plotted by connecting the points obtained from ANN model results at different model thresholds as shown in Figure 11.1. A ROC is a graph that represents a plot of *sensitivity* versus *(1 - specificity)*. The Area under ROC curve (AUROC) can be computed by the sum of trapeziums areas under the curve. An *AUROC* close to 1.0 is a considered an excellent discrimination, but a value near 0.50 suggests no discrimination (similar to a coin flip).

The ROC curve for each model was computed and compared as shown in Figure 11.1. From a visual inspection, it's clear to see that the SVM model has a more desirable accuracy due to its larger relative area under the ROC (AUROC).

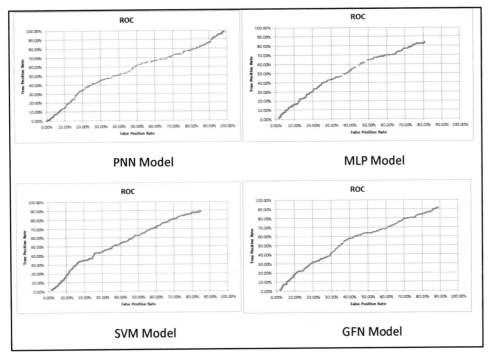

Fig. 11.1 - ROC Curves for the four ANN models

Likelihood ratio combines both sensitivity and specificity into a single measure. It provides the direct estimate of how much a test result will change the odds of having a disease. The Positive LR (LR+) shows how much the odds of the disease increase when a test is positive. The Negative LR (LR-) shows how much the odds of the disease decrease when a test is negative. Odds can be derived from probability. To convert from probability to odds, divide the probability by one minus that probability.

Positive LR is the ratio of sensitivity to one minus specificity (Delen 2009). The accuracy measures may be defined as:

$$accuracy = \frac{TP+TN}{TP+TN+FP+FN} \tag{89}$$

$$sensitivity = \frac{TP}{TP+FN} \tag{90}$$

$$specificity = \frac{TN}{TN+FP} \tag{91}$$

$$LR+ = \frac{sensitivity}{1-specificity} = \frac{\Pr(T+|D+)}{\Pr(T+|D-)} \tag{92}$$

$$LR- = \frac{1-sensitivity}{specificity} = \frac{\Pr(T-|D+)}{\Pr(T-|D-)} \tag{93}$$

An LR+ is a ratio, equal to the probability of a person who has the disease and tested positive divided by the probability of a person who does not have the disease and tested positive. An LR- is another ratio, equal to the probability of a person who has the disease and tested negative divided by the probability of a person who does not have the disease and tested negative.

Likelihood ratio is useful when the pre-test odds of having a disease are known. Then, the post-test odds of disease can be computed by:

$$odds_{post-test} = odds_{pretest} * likelihood\ ratio \tag{94}$$

This calculation is based on Bayes Theorem. One can convert odds to probability simply by (95).

$$Probability_{pretest} = \frac{(TP+FN)}{Total\ Sample}$$

Alternatively,

$$Odds_{pretest} = \frac{(Probability_{pretest})}{(1-Probability_{pretest})} \tag{95}$$

When a model uses continuous data measurements, then different thresholds may be applied in order to decide which value is the cut-off to distinguish between patients with disease. The best model has the highest values for sensitivity and specificity. In certain situations, both may not be equally important. For example, a false-negative (FN) prediction might be more critical than a false-positive (FP) prediction. If no preference is given to either measurement then, Youden's index (J) may be used to choose an appropriate cut-off, computed by (Bewick, Cheek, Ball 2004).

When using ANN models to make a binary prediction the result is a continuous measure that varies from 0.00 to 1.00. The ideal threshold that would classify patients into disease or healthy can be set using the Youden's index J. At the point where Youden's index is highest, the threshold can be set at that level. The Youden's index for each of the four ANN models were computed and used to determine the ideal threshold. The relationship between Youden's index J and sensitivity and specificity is defined as:

$$J = sensitivity + specificity - 1 \tag{95}$$

Higher value of J is desired. The maximum value that J can take is 1, when the test is perfect.

PPV corresponds to the number of true positives divided by the sum of true positives and false positives. NPV is computed as the ratio of

$$PPV = \frac{True\ Positives}{(True\ Positives + False\ Positives)} \tag{96}$$

$$NPV = \frac{True\ Negatives}{(True\ Negatives + False\ Negatives)} \tag{97}$$

Figure 11.2 shows a statistical truth table (Also known as Confusion Matrix) that illustrates how sensitivity, specificity, PPV and NPV are related. In this figure, results of the GFN model are used only as illustration to show how PPV, NPV, Sensitivity and Specificity are calculated.

		Truth (Condition) as determined by "Gold Standard"		
		Positive Condition	**Negative Condition**	
Test Outcome	Test Outcome: **Positive**	**True Positive** (TP) = 129 $1 - \beta$	**False Positive** (FP) = 336 (Type I error) A	Positive Predictive value = $$\frac{\sum True\ Positive}{\sum Test\ Outcome\ Positive}$$ = TP/(TP+FP) =129/(129+336) **=27.7%**
	Test Outcome: **Negative**	**False Negative** (FN) = 96 (Type II error) β	**True Negative** (TN) = 512 $1 - \alpha$	Negative Predictive value = $$\frac{\sum True\ Negative}{\sum Test\ Outcome\ Negative}$$ =TN/(FN+TN) =512/(96+512) **=84.2%**
		Sensitivity $$\frac{\sum True\ Positive}{\sum Condition\ Positive}$$ =TP/(TP+FN) =129/(129+96) **=57.3%**	**Specificity** $$\frac{\sum True\ Negative}{\sum Condition\ Negative}$$ =TN/(FP+TN) =512/(336+512) **=60.4%**	

Fig. 11.2 - Statistics Truth Table (Confusion Matrix)

In statistics and Medicine, Gold Standard Test refers to a diagnostic test that is best available to diagnose or classify a patient into either disease or normal condition. Gold standard test is not necessary a perfect test, but one that offers the most accurate test possible without restrictions. The ideal Gold standard test offers 100% sensitivity and specificity. In practice, however, a Gold Standard test is less accurate. For example, to diagnose brain tumor, one can perform a biopsy or an MRI. A biopsy test is regarded as the Gold Standard for diagnosing brain tumor, but since MRI test is less accurate but a practical substitute, it's regarded as an "imperfect gold standard" or "Alloyed gold standard" (Spiegelman, Schneeweiss, McDermott, 1996). Gold standard tests vary over time for each disease as the state-of-the art methods of diagnostic tests improve over time.

11.3 Comparison of results

All four models were optimized for classification of cases into a dichotomous dependent variable: the presence or absence of DVT. The results showed that the SVM algorithm was most accurate followed by the MLP model and the General feed-forward neural network model. All four methods are compared using the accuracy measurements in Table 11.1.

Table 5.1 - Accuracy Measures of Neural network models

Measurement	Probabilistic Neural Network	Support Vector Machine	Multi-Layer Perceptron-LM	Generalized Feed-forward-LM
Accuracy	0.6766	0.6673	0.6757	0.5974
Sensitivity	0.4178	0.4356	0.4000	0.5733
Specificity	0.7453	0.7288	0.7488	0.6038
LR+	1.6402	1.6059	1.5925	1.4470
LR-	0.7812	0.7745	0.8013	0.7067
Youden's J	0.1631	0.1643	0.1488	0.1771
PPV	0.3032	0.2988	0.2970	0.2777
NPV	0.8283	0.8295	0.8247	0.8421
AUC	0.5593	0.5945	0.5760	0.4176

All four models exhibited low sensitivity measures indicating their poor ability to detect true positives. This is due to the lower number of positive DVT cases in this study (only 225 out of 1,073 cases had positive DVT cases). AUC is regarded as a better measure of performance than accuracy (Ling, Huang, Zhang 2003). Since the AUC value of SVM algorithm is highest among all four ANN algorithms, one can declare that in this instance only, the SVM algorithm has highest accuracy on this data set.

11.4 Use of Oracle Program in Multi-model Analytics Framework

Since their introduction in 1960's, various neural network algorithms have been proposed and successfully implemented to classify and predict future state of output variables. Certain models are more suitable to specific class of problems based on the type and number inputs and output classifications. Typically, no single neural network model is best for all types of problem.

An approach that uses an ensemble of prognostic algorithms is shown to be effective in providing more accurate prediction (Hu, Youn & Wang 2010).

In this framework five different ensemble methods were employed for the oracle to select from. The first ensemble used conditional logic to maximize the number of TP and minimize the number of FP predictions. Studies have shown that the Area Under Characteristic (AUC) is a better measurement of an algorithm's performance than comparing Accuracy measure (Ling, Huang, Zhang 2003). The oracle program compares the AUC values for all ensembles and ANN algorithms and selects the model or ensemble with the highest AUC value. The oracle program was written in R, an open source statistical program (Wang 2012). The program was tested to evaluate and compute AUC for all ensembles.

The results of the ensembles are shown in Table 11.2. A comparison of accuracy for these ensembles appears in Table 13.

Table 11.2 - Results of the five ensemble programs

Ensemble	Schema	TP	FP	TN	FN	Total
Ensemble#1	Uses Relative preference for the more accurate model	152	426	422	73	1073
Ensemble#2	Uses TP ratio to increase TP count	105	246	602	120	1073
Ensemble#3	Reduces FN by a ratio of each model's FN count	131	345	503	94	1073
Ensemble#4	Diversity based to increase robustness	152	428	420	73	1073
Ensemble#5	Optimization based to reduce overall error	139	387	461	86	1073

Ensemble#1 took a preference ratio of four models to produce a more accurate prediction with emphasis to reduce FN count. The second ensemble combined weighted sum of predictions from each model in the ensemble. The weights were determined to maximize the number of TP predictions. Ensemble#5 selected weights by using the optimization method. The optimization model was computed using Excel Solver with one minimum objective function and five constraints. The optimum weights were 0.0, 0.03652, 0.5234, 0.437368 computed for PNN, SVM, MLP and GFN models respectively.

A comparison of accuracy measures among the five ensembles are shown in Table 11.3. One method to compare all four models and the five ensemble programs is to use the Receiver Operating Curve (ROC) plot. The ROC curve is a plot of *sensitivity* versus *(1 – specificity)*, and generally is considered a good accuracy measure of binary classifiers (Bourdes, Ferrieres, Amar, Amelineau, et al, 2011).

Table 61.3 - Comparison of Five Ensemble accuracy

Measurement	Ensemble #1	Ensemble #2	Ensemble #3	Ensemble #4	Ensemble #5
Accuracy	0.5350	0.6589	0.5909	0.5331	0.5592
Sensitivity	0.6756	0.4667	0.5822	0.6756	0.6178
Specificity	0.4976	0.7099	0.5932	0.4953	0.5436
LR+	1.3448	1.6087	1.4311	1.3385	1.3537
LR -	0.6520	0.7513	0.7043	0.6551	0.7031
Youden's J	0.1732	0.1766	0.1754	0.1708	0.1614
PPV	0.2630	0.2991	0.2752	0.2621	0.2621
NPV	0.8525	0.8338	0.8425	0.8540	0.8428
AUC	0.6035	0.6047	0.6046	0.6040	0.5943

Figure 11.3 shows a bar chart graph of AUC value for all models. The best prediction method would result in the higher AUC value.

The diagram illustrates two observations: The prediction results are not as accurate as one would like. This is attributed to the fact there were too few positive cases in the entire population to help train a more accurate predictive model. Furthermore, several of input variables were highly correlated such that the predictive contribution of some variables was less significant for making a more accurate prediction. However, prediction accuracy was improved using ensemble of models. In this particular data set, Ensemble #2 provides the highest level of AUC. Therefore, the oracle program would select Ensemble #2, for predicting DVT for patients in this situation. However, as new data arrives and the models get retrained or for other diseases and data sets, it's completely plausible that other ensembles would perform better than Ensemble#2. The point of this investigation is to emphasize that the ensemble of algorithms produces better accuracy and more robustness to predict from various data sets and for different diseases.

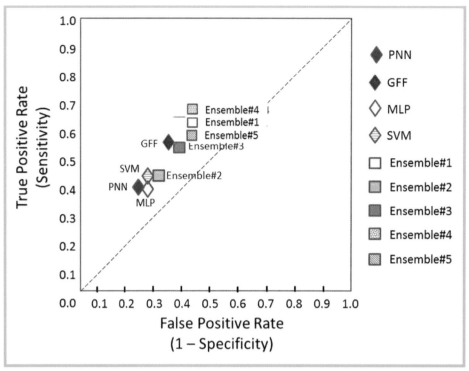

Fig. 11.3 – Comparison of Sensitivity vs. (1-Specificity) illustrating the improvement by Ensemble models

The oracle program was written in R, an open source statistical program (Wang 2012). The source code for the oracle is shown in Appendix E. R is a statistical language for analytics. It can run both in interactive and script file environments. This finding suggests that ensembles that optimize weights of combined models can drastically improve accuracy as each model contributes its best characteristics towards predicting the outcome.

A review of the results shown in tables 11.2 and 11.3 reveals that all ensemble models except for Ensemble#5 were more accurate than each neural network model alone, based on criteria established by the ensembles. The ensemble approach as demonstrated in this case study provides various schema that can improve robustness and accuracy of multiple neural networks. The results obtained in this framework illustrate the notion that multi-model frameworks can be enhanced by using various ensemble (or committee network) constructs.

11.5 Conclusions

In this clinical intelligence framework, the viability and feasibility of a prognostics and health management methods using multi-model analytics and an oracle program to predict medical disease were examined. Several rubrics for comparing accuracy model and building ensembles to enhance accuracy were developed and explained. The performance of these models varies depending on the type and volume of input and output variables. Since no single model is a perfect fit for all types of prediction, and since each of the four models had certain strengths and weaknesses. It was demonstrated that by combining multiple models one can improve classification accuracy. As was approved by the Committee, an oracle program was constructed to select the best weighted combination of results from multiple neural network models in order to enhance prediction accuracy.

This framework explored and confirmed viability of the framework in 3 ways: 1) It developed a multi-model ANN prognostics engine, 2) It developed a mechanism for comparing accuracy of multiple ANN models, and 3) It devised an oracle program to select the most accurate ensemble. The viability of the framework was evaluated and tested using a realistic retrospective dataset of 1,073 patients. Four ANN models were developed and their predictions were compared with the actual patient disease condition. Five ensembles were formed to further demonstrate that accuracy can improve by combining results of multiple ANN models.

This framework proposed and demonstrated that predictive frameworks based on multiple ANN models are viable and practical methods to patient disease prediction. It was further demonstrated through a case study that an oracle program or an overseer can select a more accurate prediction from among multiple models or multiple ensemble of models. Five different ensemble schemes were developed and the overseer "oracle" program were demonstrated as part of this framework. To demonstrate application of this framework, the ensemble model was applied to a case study to predict patients with propensity to develop DVT/PE were presented. The accuracy in terms of specificity, sensitivity and AUROC improved using the framework of multi-model algorithm approach and the oracle program. This completes the case study application of the framework.

The opportunities to apply big data analytics to clinical and business intelligence data are tremendous. Data is the new gold and we'll see the growth of analytics applications to structured and un-structured data. The future will be bright as we shine light on our data. This framework is a starting point to apply analytics to other adjacent fields in clinical intelligence including life sciences applications such as precision medicine.

Appendix A: Prognostics Methods

Prognostics models can be classified into three general types (Eklund 2009; Hines 2009; Peysson et al. 2009). Type I is reliability based. It applies the traditional time to failure analysis by tracking a population of failures and using statistical methods for the estimation of reliability. Some typical life distributions that are used in this type of prognostics include Weibull, exponential and normal distributions. Type I prognostic methods does not incorporate the real time monitoring of operating conditions or environmental conditions. For example, a system that has operated under harsher environments is likely to fail faster than the system based on past environmental conditions or the past data.

The Weibull model is frequently used in type I methods because it offers flexible distributions for a variety of failure rate profiles. The two parameter Weibull model uses a shape parameter β, and a characteristic life parameter ϑ. The result at time t is:

$$\lambda(t) = \frac{\beta}{\theta} \left(\frac{t}{\theta}\right)^{\beta-1} \tag{98}$$

Type I prognostic methods does not incorporate the real time, operating conditions or environment. For example, consider the life expectancy of a computer disk drive. The disk drive is known to have a failure distribution of 20,000 hours and standard deviation of 5,000 hours. A disadvantage of type I approach is that it does not consider the operating condition of the system. In addition, type I prognostics offers an average for failure rate but specific failure predictions are preferable. For example, a system that has operated under harsher environments is likely to fail faster than the mean time to failure (MTTF) for that system.

Type II methods are also known as the stressor-based approaches that consider the operational and environmental condition data. Type II methods can be used if the condition data are measurable and correlated to the system degradation. This approach includes methods such shock models and use traditional Markov methods. While this type of analysis is superior to Type I methods, it still lacks the unit-to-unit variance. This type considers the failures of a system in its operating environment to provide an average remaining life of a component. Some of the environmental data might include temperature, vibration, humidity and load. As an example, the proportional hazard model is a type II prognostic model. Knowing the causes, one can predict reliability of a system. The simplest model in this approach is the regression model: given the operating and environmental conditions, one can predict the system failure and remaining useful life by a regression equation:

$$Failure\ rate =$$
$$\beta_0 + \beta_1 \times Cause_1 + \beta_2 \times Cause_2 + \cdots + \beta_n \times Cause_n \tag{99}$$

The other commonly used Type II model is the Proportional Hazards Model (PHM). This model takes the environmental conditions (termed z_j) into account to modify the baseline hazard rate $\lambda_0(t)$ to produce a new hazard rate:

$$\lambda(t;z) = \lambda_0(t)e^{\left(\Sigma_{j=1}^{q}\beta_j z_j\right)} \tag{100}$$

The term z_j is a multiplicative factor, an explanatory variable or covariance that explains the effect on failure rate. The parameter $\lambda_0(t)$ is an arbitrary baseline hazard function and β_j is a model parameter (Eklund 2009).

As an example, the proportional hazard model is a type II prognostic model. Using the disk drive example, one can determine the expected failure rate if the disk drive's total operating hours to date and the disk drive's prior operating condition such as historical temperatures and number of disk accesses are known. These models are usually cause and effect based.

Type III prognostic methods are condition-based, namely they characterize the lifetime of a system in operation in its specific environment. They estimate the remaining life of a specific component or the entire system. Among methods used in Type III prognostics are the General Path Model (GPM), Neural Network models, Expert systems, Fuzzy rule-based systems, and multi-state analysis. Another example of type III model is the cumulative Damage model.

One of the prognostic models that can gather and learn failure parameter data is Artificial Neural Networks (ANN) and is discussed next in this paper. As sensors become smaller and smarter, the proliferation of sensors implies increasing volume of data that can be processed for prognostics. ANNs are ideal constructs for medical prognostics because they can model feed-forward systems, compute non-linear relationships and analyze very large number of input data. In fact, given their parallel architecture, ANNs can function or even substitute for missing data. They are able to learn the inherent rules in a given system, can maintain long term memory and discern patterns even in noisy and changing environments. Because of these characteristics, ANNs are increasingly selected for prognostics studies and this is a reason that I've selected ANNs for This framework.

The cumulative damage model tracks the irreversible accumulation of damage in systems or components. The statistical cumulative damage model considers the number of possible damage states and a transition matrix (for representing a multi-state Markov Chain) to provide a damage prediction for multiple cyclical loads.

Another type III method is the Shock model. This approach is used to predict the RUL for a system subject to randomly arriving shocks. The shocks deliver certain damage of random magnitude to the system. These models are continuous in time and consequently, the degradation measures are also continuous. Shock models are estimated from historical failure data. They are similar to the Markov Chain model, except that the time between shocks and the shock magnitudes are continuous and random variables.

GPM models were proposed in 1993 as a statistical method for estimating a time-to-failure distribution using degradation measures. GPM models assume that the degradation of a system is a function of time, duty cycle or some other measure. The model extrapolates a degradation function to predict RUL. GPM makes two assumptions: A) Each individual device (or system) has a unique degradation signal and B) The failure occurs at a critical threshold. This model starts with a parametric model to the exemplar degradation paths. It then computes the mean and covariance values to explain individual random parameters. It can use Bayesian probability functions to modify the posterior RUL values from apriori data. It extrapolates the critical failure threshold to estimate RUL.

The reliability and survival analysis techniques, both parametric and non-parametric methods are noteworthy of discussion. These methods as will be discussed later can be applied to prognostics. Finally, there is the Artificial Neural Network (ANN) models that are used for this framework and will be explained in more detail later in this paper. A synthesis of how these methods compare and their suitability to predicting clinical patient status will be presented.

Reliability and Predictive Analytics:

Reliability is defined as the probability that product will perform its intended function, satisfactorily for its intended life when operating under specified condition (Kapur 2010). A clinical definition can be derived from this technical description; Reliability is the probability that a patient will not develop certain medical complication during the length stay under medical care of the care provider(s). Reliability is measured by several indicators such as Mean Time Between Failure (MTBF), Failure rate and Percentiles of Life. Each measurement can be computed from corresponding equations that are derived from empirical and statistical distribution functions.

In general, Reliability at time t, is shown as *R(t)*. Failures are measured by *f(t)*, the probability density function for the time of failure, a random variable T. The cumulative distribution function for random variable *T* is shown by *F(t)*. Thus, one can write the following expressions to define *F(t)*, *f(t)* and *R(t)*:

$$F(t) = P\,[T \leq t] = \int_0^t f(\tau)d\tau \tag{101}$$

$$f(t) = \frac{dF(t)}{dt} \tag{102}$$

$$R(t) = 1 - F(t) \tag{103}$$

Additional treatment of Reliability can be found from text by Kapur and Lamberson (Kapur, Lamberson 1977).

Appendix B: A Neural Network Example

Consider the following classification problem as described in section 2. Suppose we're considering classifying patients by only four input variables, Glucose (G), Body mass (M), Systolic Blood pressure (S) and Platelet count (P):

Values for G, M, S, and P for past patients are given for the model to train on, as listed below. The first step in classification is to normalize the input data to unit length. Normalizing to unit length implies that the sum of squares of values in a given data set are equal to 1. This technique was explained in section 4.2.

The classification problem is defined as follows. There are two sets of data vectors: one set of data vectors belong to the TRUE set (Patients with DVT) and another set belongs to the FALSE set (No DVT cases). A new patient with the normalized data is introduced and the goal is to classify that patient with the normalized values of: [0.75, 0.32, 0.60, 0.21].

The previously classified data sets and their corresponding new normalized values are computed as follows:

[117, 194, 140, 276] , DVT = TRUE, normalized: [0.31, 0.51, 0.37, 0.72]

[120, 164, 213, 315] , DVT = TRUE, normalized: [0.27, 0.38, 0.49, 0.73]

[115, 145, 170, 288] , DVT = TRUE, normalized: [0.30, 0.38, 0.44, 0.75]

[122, 165, 155, 290] , DVT = TRUE, normalized: [0.31, 0.43, 0.40, 0.75]

For patients with no DVT outcome:

[122, 144, 110, 236] , DVT = FALSE, normalized: [0.38, 0.45, 0.34, 0.73]

[140, 154, 153, 176] , DVT = FALSE, normalized: [0.45, 0.49, 0.49, 0.56]

[145, 135, 130, 218] , DVT = FALSE, normalized: [0.45, 0.42, 0.40, 0.68]

[132, 155, 115, 190] , DVT = FALSE, normalized: [0.44, 0.51, 0.38, 0.63]

The following kernel for computing PNN pattern and summation based on derivations from Equations (39) and (41):

$$z_A = f_A(x) = \sum_{i=1}^{N_k} e^{\frac{(x^t w_{ki} - 1)}{\sigma^2}}$$

The new patient with the normalized data set of [0.75, 0.32, 0.60, 0.21] is to be classified. In this example, it's assumed that σ is equal to 1.0 for sake of simplifying calculations. Next, it's possible to compute $f_A(x)$ for each data set:

.31*.75+.51*.32+.37*.60+.72*.21 − 1.0 = -0.239   exp (-0.239) = 0.787

exp (-0.220) = 0.803

exp (-0.228) = 0.796

exp (-0.231) = 0.794

Sum1 = 3.180

Similarly for the second class, it's possible to compute:

.38*.75+.45*.32+.34*.60+.73*.21 – 1.0 = -0.213   exp (-0.213) = 0.808

exp (-0.095) = 0.910

exp (-0.144) = 0.866

exp (-0.145) = 0.865

Sum2 = 3.449

Since Sum2 > Sum1, it implies that the data points for this patient are closer to FALSE classification as the sum of values associated with the FALSE class is higher. Thus this patient belongs to the FALSE classification and is predicted to have DVT=FALSE (i.e. prognostics for DVT is negative).

Appendix C: Back Propagation Algorithm Derivation

In general, there are two types of learning processes: the batch mode and the sequential mode. On the conditions for these mathematical calculations is that the function $\varphi_j\left(v_j(n)\right)$ must be continuous and differentiable so one can obtain $\varphi_j'(v_j(n))$. Also the choice of η as the learning rate is important to be set at the appropriate value. The backward propagation is an approximation to the steepest descent algorithm. If the researcher uses a small η there is risk of getting unstable results. Rumelhart (Rumelhart 1986) suggested adding a momentum value to the learning rate η according to this algorithm:

Case 1: If $\frac{\partial E(n)}{\partial w_{ji}(n)}$ has the same sign for all n, then one can say that $|\Delta w_{kj}|$ grows in magnitude. This represents the case of an accelerated descent.

Case 2: If in contrast $\frac{\partial E(n)}{\partial w_{ji}(n)}$ alternates its sign in every iteration, then $|\Delta w_{kj}|$ is small in magnitude and more controllable than the first case. The momentum term is significant because it accelerates learning but also help to avoid local optima.

The Back propagation algorithm employs the following eight steps. This is adapted from Zurada (Zurada 1997) and Sengupta (Sengupta 2009):

Given p training pairs shown by: $\{z_1, d_1, z_2, d_2, \dots, z_P, d_P\}$,

where z_i is a (I X 1), d_i is (K X 1), and i= 1, 2, …, P.

Step 1: Choose > 0, E_{max} . Weights W and V are initialized at small random values. W is (K X J), V is (J X 1). Initialize q, p and E:

$$q \leftarrow 1, p \leftarrow 1, E \leftarrow 0$$

Step 2: Start training. Input is presented and the layers' outputs are computed using $\Delta w_i = cf(w_i^t\, x)x$:

$$z \leftarrow z_p, \qquad d \leftarrow d_p$$

$$y_j \leftarrow f\left(V_j^t z\right), for\ j = 1, \dots, J$$ Where V_j is a column vector and is the jth row of V, and

$$o_k \leftarrow f\left(W_k^t y\right), for\ k = 1, \dots, K$$ Where W_k is a column vector and is the kth row of W.

Step 3: Compute the Error value by comparing the desired output versus network output:

$$E \leftarrow E + \frac{1}{2}\,(d_k - o_k)^2\ for\ k = 1, \dots, K.$$

Step 4: Compute error signal vectors δ_o and δ_y of both layers. Vector δ_o is (K X 1) and δ_y is (J X 1). The error signal terms of the output layer in this step are:

$$\delta_{ok} = \frac{1}{2}\,[(d_k - o_k)(1 - \delta_k^2)]\quad for\ k = 1, \dots, K$$

The error signal terms of the hidden layer in this step are computed by:

$$\delta_{yj} = \frac{1}{2}(1 - y_j^2) \sum_{k=1}^{K} \delta_{ok} w_{kj}, \text{ for } j=1, \ldots, J$$

Step 5: Adjust the output layer weights by:

$$w_{kj} = w_{kj} + \eta \delta_{ok} y_j \text{ for } k = 1, \ldots, K \text{ and } j = 1, \ldots, J$$

Step 6: Adjust the hidden layer weights:

$$V_{ji} = V_{ji} + \eta \delta_{yj} z_i \text{ for } i = 1, \ldots, I \text{ and } j = 1, \ldots, J$$

Step 7: If $p < P$ then increment p and q: $q \leftarrow q + 1, p \leftarrow p + 1$, go to step 2, otherwise go to step 8.

Step 8: The training cycle is completed. If $E < E_{max}$ the training session is finished. The weights are defined by W, V, q and E. If $E > E_{max}$ then $p \leftarrow 1, E \leftarrow 0$ and initiate a new training cycle by going to step 2.

Most recently, practitioners prefer other algorithms such as the Conjugate Gradient Descent and Simulated Annealing (Masters 2005) to backward propagation. These algorithms offer faster convergence to learning. Conjugate Gradient Descent is a deterministic optimization method that attempts to find local minimum of a function. Simulated Annealing is designed to ensure that the training algorithm overcomes getting trapped in local minima.

Appendix D: NeuroSolutions Software Description

In this framework, four different commercial software packages for neural network modeling were evaluated. The evaluation considered several criteria for selection. The packages were compared on the following criteria:

- A large library of ANN algorithms
- Ability to combine multiple algorithms
- Robustness of the software on large data sets so it would be stable and not crash
- Ability to measure accuracy and provide accuracy measurements for each model
- Ability to use Excel input data files
- Ability to export (or package) the model for external use

This evaluation included building actual models using the DVT/PE case study and learning the pros and cons of each package. Of the four models evaluated, a commercial neural network software entitled NeuroSolutions™ was employed for building all ANN models. NeuroSolutions is an object-oriented environment for neural networks that implements both static and dynamic, arbitrary, user-defined topologies, which can be adapted with the most popular learning paradigms. NeuroSolutions is developed, supported and licensed by NeuroDimension, Incorporated, Gainesville, Florida.

The graphical user interface uses the electronic design metaphor for neural network design, in which neural "components" are placed on a "breadboard" and interconnected with each other. The component icons are associated univocally with the objects that implement the functionality of the package. The interface is built with the idea of showing to the user all the important variables that pertain to the configuration of the components.

Adaptive systems can be better understood if all the internal variables and parameters can be visualized. For this reason, NeuroSolutions includes an extensive set of graphical probes.

NeuroSolutions can implement a wide array of models including linear regression models, nonlinear regression models, multilayer perceptrons (MLPs) with arbitrary topologies, radial basis function networks, digital filters, time lagged networks of arbitrary topologies, recurrent networks of arbitrary topologies, associative memories, support vector machines, neuro-fuzzy, principal (and nonlinear) component networks, competitive and Kohonen networks. It implements several types of backpropagation to train static and recurrent networks (static backpropagation, fixed point learning, backpropagation thought time), several cost functions (L1, L2, Linf norms). It implements several types of search procedures (momentum learning, delta-bar-delta, conjugate gradient and Fahlman's quickprop), and enables the mixing of any one of these models.

The package is a very open development environment in that it enables the user to extend the basic components by modifying the default C code and compiling the new components as DLLs (Dynamic Link Libraries).

NeuroSolutions for Neural Network Control

NeuroSolutions is an ideal environment for developing neural control systems for a number of reasons. Its icon-based graphical user interface and extensive probing capabilities provides a rapid prototyping environment for experimenting with various neural network architectures and algorithms. If a desired algorithm is not included with the package, then a custom one can be easily implemented by writing Dynamic Link Libraries (DLLs) to override the functionality of the default neural components.

NeuroSolutions has an extensive API library (Application Programming Interface) that makes it fully accessible from external programs. Once the neural network is designed, an automated test procedure could be written to feed the neural network the input data and extract the output data. This data could reside on the local file system or it could come from an external source which is interfaced to one of the computer's I/O ports.

The final stage of building the control system is to deploy the neural network to the actual control environment. NeuroSolutions allows you to encapsulate a specific neural network design by automatically generating the core (non-graphical) C++ source code for it. This C++ code can then be embedded into the code for the digital control program or compiled as a self-contained object such as a dynamic link library (DLL).

NeuroSolutions currently implements an impressive array of first order search techniques (gradient, momentum, adaptive step sizes (two different methods), annealed step size, independent step size) and an optimal line search algorithm called – Conjugate Gradient.

NeuroDimension, Inc. was founded in 1991, in Gainesville, Florida, by medical and computer engineering specialists whose original goal was to develop software tools that would improve their own efficiency and productivity. NeuroDimension's first product, NeuroSolutions v1.0, was released in 1994. Since that time there have been numerous enhancements to NeuroSolutions and several new products have been released (NeuroSolutions for Excel, Custom Solution Wizard, Genetic Server, and TradingSolutions), resulting in continuous sales and personnel growth.

Appendix E: The Oracle Program

The oracle program is the overseer module that selects the Ensemble with the highest value of AUC. The oracle program was written in R, an open source statistical package (Wang 2012) and was tested on the 1,073 data sets and all Ensembles. The source codes is listed below. The program computes the AUC for each ANN algorithm and Ensembles compared to the actual truth (presence or absence of disease) for prior data. The first column is the actual truth and the subsequent columns are the data for ANN algorithms and Ensembles.

```
#########################################
###### R code for computing AUC     ######
###### Peter Ghavami – Adapted      ######
######    From Wang 2012            ######
#########################################


### Load library packages ###

install.packages("verification")
library(verification)


### Import the input data file ###

## select the data file in the pop out window
data<-read.csv(file.choose(),header=T)  # Import data from csv file


### Purpose: write a R function to compute AUC ###
### function name: getAUC
### function input:
###     D: true disease status
###     T: continuous test results of ANN and Ensembles
### function output: AUC value for this test

getAUC<-function(D, T){
roc.area(D, T)$A
}                               # Call the getAUC function.


### compute the AUC values for each test in the data

### result for MLP
getAUC(data[,1],data[,2])       #MLP data is in the 2nd column

### result for PNN
getAUC(data[,1],data[,6])       #PNN data is in the 6th column
```

```
### result for GFF
getAUC(data[,1],data[,10])          #GFF data is in the 10th column

### result for SVM
getAUC(data[,1],data[,14])          #SVM data is in the 14th column

### result for Ensemble1
getAUC(data[,1],data[,18])          #Ensemble1 data is in the 18th column

### result for Ensemble2
getAUC(data[,1],data[,22])          #Ensemble2 data is in the 22nd column

### result for Ensemble3
getAUC(data[,1],data[,26])          #Ensemble3 data is in the 22nd column

### result for Ensemble4
getAUC(data[,1],data[,30])          #Ensemble4 data is in the 30th column

### result for Ensemble5
getAUC(data[,1],data[,34])          #Ensemble5 data is in the 34th column
```

References:

(Aamodt, Plaza 1994). Aamodt, A., Plaza, E., Case-Based Reasoning: Foundational Issues, Methodological Variations, and System Approaches , *AI Communications, Vol, 7, Nr. 1*, March 1994.

(Adams, Wert 2005) Adams, J. B., Wert, Y., "Logistic and Neural Network Models for Predicting a Hospital Admission", Journal of Applied Statistics, Vol. 32, No. 8, 861-869, 2005

(Allison 1995). Allison, P. D., *Survival Analysis using the SAS system*, SAS Institute publication, 1995, Cary, NC.

(AMA 2010). CPT 2011 Professional Edition, Michelle Abraham, *American Medical Association*, American Medical Association Press, Oct 20, 2010.

(Arthi, Tamilarasi 2008). Arthi, K., Tamilarasi, A., Prediction of autistic disorder using neuro fuzzy systems by applying ANN technique, *International Journal of Developmental Neuroscience, 26 (2008)* 699-704

(Baxt 1991). Baxt, W. G., *Use of an Artificial Neural Network for the Diagnosis of Myocardial Infarction*. Annals of Internal Medicine, Dec 1, 1991, Vol. 115, no. 11, pg 843-848

(Bewick, Cheek, Ball 2004) Bewick, V., Cheek, L., Ball, J., "Statistics review 13: Receiver operating characteristic curves", *Critical Care*, Vol. 8, no. 6, December 2004

(Blount, Ebling, Eklund, James, et al. 2010) Blount, M., Ebling, M. R., Eklund, J. M. , James, A. G. , McGregor, C ., Percival, N. , Smith, K. P., and Sow, D. (2010). Real-time Analysis for Intensive Care. Development and Deployment of the Artemis Analytic System. *IEEE Engineering in Medicine and Biology Magazine,* March/April 2010

(Bourdes, et al 2011) Bourdes, V., Ferrieres, J., Amar, J., Amelineau, E., Bonnevay, S., Berlion, M., Danchin, N., "Prediction of persistence of combined evidence-based cardiovascular medications in patients with acute coronary syndrome after hospital discharge using neural networks", *Medical & Biological Engineering Computing*, 49:947-955, 2011

(Bottaci, Drew, Hartley, Hadfield, et al. 1997). Bottaci, L., Drew, P. J., Hartley, J. E., Hadfield, M. B., Farouk, R., Lee, P. WR., Macintyre, I. MC., Duthie, G. S., Monson, J. RT. (1996). Artificial Neural Networks Applied to Outcome Prediction for Colorectal Cancer Patients in Separate Institutions. *The Lancet, Vol. 350, Issue 9076*, Aug 16, 1997, Pg 469-472

(Breiman, Friedman, Olshen, Stone 1984) L. Breiman, J.H. Friedman, R.A. Olshen, C.J. Stone, *Classification and regression trees*. Monterey, CA: Wadsworth & Brooks/Cole Advanced Books & Software, 1984.

(Brown, Strong, 2001). Brown, S.W., Strong, V., The use of seizure-alert dogs, *Seizure, 2001, 10*:39-41.

(CEBM 2012). Center for Evidence Based Medicine website, EBM Tools, http://www.cebm.net/index.aspx?o=1023 , accessed, March 22, 2012

(Coble, Hines 2009). Coble, J., Hines, J. W., Identifying Optimal Prognostic Parameters from Data: A Genetic Algorithms Approach, *Annual Conference of the Prognostics and Health Management Society*, 2009

(Coble, Hines 2009). Coble, J., Hines, J. W., Fusing Data Sources for Optimal Prognostic Parameter Selection,

Sixth American Nuclear Society International Topical Meeting on Nuclear Plant Instrumentation, Control, and Human-Machine Interface Technologies NPIC & HMIT 2009, Knoxville, Tennessee, April 5-9, 2009

(Collett 1994). Collett, D., *Modeling survival data in medical research*. London: Chapman & Hall.

(Daley, Narayanan, Leffler 2010). Daley, M., Narayanan, N., Leffler, C. W., Model-derived assessment of cerebrovascular resistance and cerebral blood flow following traumatic brain injury, *Experimental Biology and Medicine, Vol 235*, April 2010

(Davenport, Dennis, Wellwood, Warlow 1996) Davenport, R.J., Dennis, M.S., Wellwood, I., Warlow, C., "Complications after acute stroke", *Stroke*, Vo. 27, pg 415-420, 1996

(Dayhoff, DeLeo 2001). Dayhoff, J. E., DeLeo, J. M., Artificial Neural Networks, Opening the Black Box. *Cancer 2001; 19*:1615-35. Presented at the Conference on Prognostic Factors and Staging in Cancer Management: Contributions of Artificial Neural Networks and Other Statistical Methods.

(Delen 2009) Delen, D., "Analysis of cancer data: a data mining approach", *Expert Systems*, February 2009, Vol. 26, No. 1

(Dictionary.com 2012). www.Dictionary.com, online, an IAC company, Accessed, Jan 2012.

(Doyle, Francis, Tannenbaum 1990). Doyle, J., Francis, B., Tannenbaum, A., *Feedback Control Theory*, Macmillan Publishing Co, 1990.

(Dybowski, Grant, Weller, Chang 1996). Dybowski, R., Gant, V., Weller, P., and Chang, R., Prediction of Outcome in Critically ill Patients Using Artificial Neural Network Synthesised by Genetic Algorithm. *The Lancet, Vol 347, Issue 9009*, April 27, 1996, pg 1146-1150

(Eklund 2009). Eklund, N. H.W., Prognostics and Health Management - Part 1: Data Driven Anomaly Detection & Diagnosis, *Annual Conference of the Prognostics and Health Management Society*, Diagnostics Tutorials, 2009

(Floyd, Lo Yun, Sullivan, et al 1994). Floyd, C. E., Lo, J. Y., Yun, A. J., Sullivan, D. C., Kornguth, P. J., Prediction of Breast Cancer Malignancy Using an Artificial Neural Network. *Cancer, Vol. 74, no. 11*, Dec. 1, 1994.

(Fuller, McCullough, Bao 2009). Fuller, R. L., McCullough, E. C., Bao, M. Z., Averill, R. F., "Estimating the Costs of Potentially Preventable Hospital Acquired Complications", *Healthcare Financing Review*, Vo. 30, No. 4, Summer 2009

(Gao, Young, Ornstein, Pile-Spellman, et al. 1997). Gao, E., Young W., Ornstein, E., Pile-Spellman, J., Qiyuan, M., A theoretical model of cerebral hemodynamics: Application to the study of Arteriovenous Malformations, *Journal of Cerebral Blood Flow and Metabolism, 1997, 17*, 905-918

(Ghavami, Kapur 2011) P. Ghavami, K. Kapur, "Prognostics & Artificial Neural Network Applications in Patient Healthcare", *Proceedings of IEEE Prognostics and Health Management Conference*, June 2011

(Graunt 1662). Graunt, J., Natural and Political Observations Made Upon the Bills of Mortality.

(Hahnfeldt, Panigraphy, Folkman, Hlatkey, et al. 1999). Hahnfeldt, P., Panigraphy, D., Folkman, J., Hlatkey, L., Tumor development under angiogenic signaling: a dynamic theory of tumor growth, treatment response and postvascular dormacy, *Cancer Research 59*, 4770-4778, 1999

(Haykin 1998). Haykin, S., *Neural Networks, A Comprehensive Foundation*, 2nd Edition, Prentice Hall, 1999

(Hines 2009). Hines W. J., Empirical Methods for Process and Equipment Prognostics, *Annual Conference of the Prognostics and Health Management Society*, Prognostics Tutorials, 2009

(Hu, Youn, Wang 2010). Hu, C., Youn, B.D., Wang, P., Ensemble of data-driven prognostics algorithms with Weight Optimization and K-Fold Cross Validation, *Annual Conference of the Prognostics and Health Management (PHM) Society*, Oct 10-16 2010, Portland, OR.

(INCOSE 2000). What is a system?, Version 2.0, *INCOSE (International Council on Systems Engineering Council) Systems Engineering Handbook*, July 2000.

(Jervis, McGinn 2008) Jervis, R., McGinn, T., Evidence-based Medicine, Clinical prediction rules for hospitals, *Mount Sinai Journal of Medicine* 75: 472-477, 2008

(Kalilani, Atashili, 2006). Linda Kalilani, Julius Atashili, Measuring Additive Interaction using Odds Ratios, *Epidemiol Perspect Innov.*, 2006; 3: 5.

(Kapur 2010). Kapur, K., *Seminar on Prognostics, Dept. of Industrial & Systems Engineering, University of Washington*, Feb-March, 2010.

(Kapur, Lamberson 1997). Kapur, K., Lamberson, L. R., *Reliability in Engineering Design*, 1977

(Kimmel, Axelrod 2002). Kimmel, M., Axelrod, D.E., *Branching processes in biology*, Springer Verlag, New York, NY, 2002

(Kirton, Winter, Wirrell, Snead 2008) Kirton, A., Winter, A., Wirrell, E., Snead, O. C., "Seizure response dogs: Evaluation of a formal training program*", Epilepsy & Behavior*, 13 (2008) 499-504.

(Kodell, Pearce, Baek, et al. 2009). Kodell, R. L., Pearce, B. A., Baek, S., Moon, H., Ahn, H., A model-free ensemble method for class prediction with application to biomedical decision making, *Artificial Intelligence in Medicine (2009), 46*, 267-276

(Kon, Plaskota 2000). Kon, A., M., Plaskota, L., Complexity of Predictive Neural Networks, *International Conference on Complex Systems*, May, 2000.

(Kwakernaak, Sivan 1972). Kwakernaak, H., Sivan, R., *Linear Optimal Control Systems*, John Wiley & Sons, 1972

(Laupacis, Sekar, Stiell 1997) Laupacis, A., Sekar, N., Stiell, I. G., Clinical prediction rules. A review and suggested modifications of methodological standards. *JAMA* 1997; 277:488-94.

(Ling, Huang, Zhang 2003). Ling, C.X., Huang, J., Zhang, H., "AUC: a Statistically Consistent and more Discriminating Measure than Accuracy", *International Joint Conference on Artificial Intelligence, 2003, Vol. 18*, pages 519-526, Lawrence Erlbaum Associates, LTD.

(Ling, Huang, Zhang, 2003). Ling, C.X., Huang, J., Zhang, H., "AUC: A Better Measure than Accuracy in Comparing Learning Algorithms", *Lecture Notes in Computer Science*, 2003, ISSU 2671, pages 329-341, Springer-Verlag

(Limaye, Mastrangelo, Zerr, Jeffries 2008). Limaye, S. S., Mastrangelo, C. M., Zerr, D. M., Jeffries, H., A statistical approach to reduce hospital-associated infections, *Quality Engineering, 20*:414-425, 2008

(Linder, Geier, Kolliker 2004) Linder, R. Geier, J., Kolliker,M., "Artificial neural networks, classification trees, and regression: Which method for which customer base?" *Database Marketing & Customer Strategy Management*, Vol 11, 4, 344-356, 2004

(Lisboa, Taktak 2005). Lisboa, P. J., Taktak, A. F.G., The Use of Artificial Networks in Decision Support in Cancer: A Systematic Review. *Neural Networks, Vol 19, Issue 4*, May 2006, pg 408-415

(Macal 2005). Macal, C., Model Verification and Validation, The University of Chicago and Argonne National Laboratory, *Workshop on "Threat Anticipation: Social Science Methods and Models"*, April 7-9, 2005, Chicago, IL.

(Maguire 2007) Maguire, P., "The new crackdown on preventable complications", *Today's Hospitalist*, October 2007.

(Masters 1995). Masters, T., *Advanced Algorithms for Neural Networks: A C++ Sourcebook*, Wiley, New York, 1995

(McGinn, Guyatt, Wyer, Naylor, et al. 2000). McGinn, T. G., Guyatt, G. H., Wyer, P. C., Naylor, C. D., Stiell, I. G., Richardson, W. S., Users' Guide to Medical Literature, *JAMA 2000; 284(1)*:79-84; For the Evidence-based Medicine Working Group.

(Merriam-Webster Dictionary 2011). Merriam-Webster dictionary online, www.Merriam-webster.com/dictionary/, an Encyclopedia Britannica Company. Accessed December 2011.

(MIT 2010) See http://classics.Mit.edu/Hippocrates/ prognost.html. Date accessed: Feb 2010.

(Monterola, Lim, Garcia, Saloma 2002). Monterola, C., Lim, M., Garcia, J., Saloma, C., Feasibility of a Neural Network as Classifier of Undecided Respondents in a Public Opinion Survey, *International Journal of Public Opinion Research, Vol. 14, No. 2*, 2002

(Neuro Dimenstions, Inc 2011). NeuroDimension, Inc., Gainesville, Florida, NeuroSolutions software, Version 6.0

(NHS Casemix 2009) "The Casemix Design Framework - 2009", by Casemix Design Authority. Version 2.3, Issue Date: December 2009. The Health and Social Care Information Centre, Casemix Service.

(Niu, Yang, Pecht 2010). Niu, G., Yang, B., Pecht, M., Development of an optimized condition-based maintenance system by data fusion and reliability-centered maintenance, *Reliability Engineering and System Safety*, V95, n7, p786-796, 2010

(O'Connor, Bennett, Stacey, Barry, et al. 2009). O'Connor, A. M., Bennett, C.L., Stacey, D., Barry, M., Col, N. F., Eden, K.B., Entwistle, V. A., Fiset, V., Decision aids for people facing health treatment or screening decisions (Review), *The Cochrane Collaboration*, Wiley 2009

(Ozbay 1999). Ozbay, H., *Introduction to Feedback Control Theory*, CRC Press, 1999

(Park, Kim, Chun 2006). Park, Y., Kim, B., Chun, S., "New knowledge extraction technique using probability for case-based reasoning: application to medical diagnosis, *Expert Systems*, Feb 2006, Vol. 23, No. 1

(Pecht 2008). Pecht, M., *Prognostics and Health Management of Electronics*, Wiley 2008

(Peysson, Ouladsine, Outbib 2009). Peysson, F., Ouladsine, M. and Outbib R., Complex System Prognostics: A New Systemic Approach, *Annual Conference of the Prognostics and Health Management Society*, 2009

(Principe, Euliano, Lefebvre 1999). Principe, J. C., Euliano, N.R., Lefebvre, W.C., *Neural and Adaptive Systems, Fundamentals Through Simulations*, John Wiley & Sons, 1999

(Principe 2011). Principe, J. C., Conversations with Jose` C. Principe, University of Texas, Sept. 2011

(Prodormidis, Chan, Stolfo 2000). Prodormidis, A.L., Chan, P.K., Stolfo, S.J., Meta-learning in distributed data mining systems: Issues and Approaches, *Advances in Distributed Data Mining*, MIT Press, 2000

(Ravdin, Clark, 1992). Ravdin, P. M. and Clark, G. M., A Practical Application of Neural Network Analysis for Predicting Outcome of Individual Breast Cancer Patients. *Breast Cancer Research and Treatment, Vol. 22, No. 3*, Oct. 1992. pg 285-293

(Rumelhart, Hinton, Williams 1986). Rumelhart, D. E., Hinton, G. E., and Williams, R. J. (1986) Learning representations by back-propagating errors, *Nature, vol. 323*, pp. 533-536, 1986

(Schlimmer, Granger, Jr. 1986). Schlimmer, J.C., Granger, Jr., R.H., Incremental Learning from Noisy Data, *Machine Learning 1*:317-354, 1986, Kluwer Publishers, Boston

(Sengupta 2009). Sengupta, S., *Lecture series on Neural Networks and Applications by Prof. S. Sengupta*, Department of Electronics and Electrical Communication Engineering, Indian Institute of Technology, Kharagpur, source: NPTEL, http://nptel.iitm.ac.in , accessed 2009- 2012

(Smye, Clayton 2002). Smye, S. W., Clayton, R. H., Mathematical modeling for the new millennium: medicine by numbers, *Medical Engineering & Physics, 24 (2002)*, 565-574

(Souter 2011). Souter, M., Conversations on diagnostic markers and predictors, April 7, 2011.

(Spiegelman, Schneeweiss, McDermott, 1996). Spiegelman, D., Schneeweiss, S., McDermott, A., Measurement Error Correction for Logistic Regression Models with an "Alloyed Gold Standard", *American Journal of Epidemiology*, Vol. 145, no. 2, 1996

(Spruance, Reid, Grace, Samore 2004) Spruance, S. L., Reid, J. E., Grace, M., Samore, M., "Hazard Ratio in Clinical Trials", *Antimicrobial Agents and Chemotherapy*, Vol. 48(8), Aug 2004

(StopDVT.org 2011). www.StopDVT.org website, page accessed: http://stopdvt.org/FAQ.aspx, Accessed October 2011.

(Strong, Brown Walker 1999) Strong, V., Brown, S.W., Walker, R., "Seizure-alert dogs-fact or fiction"?, *Seizure*. 1999; 8:26-65.

(Swierniak, Kimmel, Smieja 2009)Andrezej Swierniak, Marek Kimmel, Jaroslaw Smieja, "Mathematical modeling as a tool for planning anticancer therapy", *European Journal of Pharmacology*, 625 (2009) 108-121

(Toll, Janssen, Vergouwe, Moons 2008). Toll, D. B., Janssen, K. J. M., Vergouwe, Y., Moons, K. G. M., Validation, updating and impact of clinical prediction rules: A review. *Journal of Clinical Epidemiology*, 61 (2008) 1085-1094.

(Tsai, Pollock, Brownie 2009). Tsai, K., Pollock, K., Brownie, C., "Effects of violation of assumptions for survival analysis methods in radiotelemetry studies", *Journal of Wildlife Management*, 63(4):1369-1375, 2009

(TU 1996). TU, J.V., Advantages and disadvantages of using artificial neural networks versus logistic regression for predicting medical outcomes, *Journal of Clinical Epidemiology*, 1996, Nov; 49(11): 1225-31.

(Uckun, Goebel, Lucas 2008). Uckun, S., Goebel, K. and Lucas, P. J. F., Standardizing Research Methods for Prognostics, *2008 International Conference on Prognostics and Health Management,* 2008

(Vichare, Pecht 2006). Vichare, N. M., and Pecht, M., Prognostics and Health Management of Electronics, *IEEE Transactions on Components and Packaging Technologies, Vol 29, No. 1*, March 2006.

(Virchow 1856). Virchow, R.,Virchow's Triad. Virchow's Triad was first formulated by the German physician Rudolf Virchow in 1856.

(Wang 2012). Wang, Z., Conversations about neural network algorithms and accuracy measures. Department of Biostatistics, University of Washington.

(Wang 2012). Wang, Z., Conversations and collaboration for calculating AUC using R statistical language. Department of Biostatistics, University of Washington.

(Webber, Litt, Wilson, Lesser 1994). Webber, W. R. S., Litt, B., Wilson, K., Lesser, R. P. (1994), Practical detection of epileptiform discharges (EDs) in the EEG using an artificial neural network: a comparison of raw and parameterized EEG data. *Electroencephalography and clinical Neurophysiology, 91,* 194-204

(Wells, Anderson, Bromanis, Mitchell, et al. 1997). Wells, P.S., Anderson, D.R., Bromanis, J., Guy, F., Mitchell, M., Gray, L., Clement, C., Robinson, K.S., Lewandowski, B., Value of assessment of pretest probability of deep-vein thrombosis in clinical management, *The Lancet, Vol 350, Issue 9094*, pg 1795-1798, 20 December 1997.

(WHO 2012) *Library of ICD9 and ICD10 codes*, World Health Organization's library of   International Statistical Classification   of   Diseases   and   Related   Health   Problems, http://www.who.int/classifications/icd/revision/en/index.html, accessed, March 09, 2012

(Williamoski, Chen 1999). Williamowski, B. M., Chen, Y., Efficient algorithm for Training Neural Networks with one Hidden Layer, *IEEE International Joint Conference on Neural Networks*, 1999

(Williams, Pembroke 1989). Williams, H., Pembroke, A., Sniffer dogs in the melanoma clinic?, *Lancet, 1989, 1(8640)*;734

(Wishart 1969). Wishart, D., Symposium on Control Theory, A survey of Control Theory. *Journal of the Royal Statistical Society, Series A*, Royal Statistical Society, 1969.

(Yu, Liu, McKenna, Reisner, et al. 2006). Yu, C., Liu, Z., McKenna, T., Reisner, A. T., Reifman, J., A Method for Automatic Identification of Reliable Heart Rates Calculated from ECG and PPG Waveforms, *Journal of the American Medical Informatics Association, vol. 13, No. 3*, May/Jun 2006.

(Zadeh, Desoer 1963). Zadeh, L. A., and Desoer, C., *Linear Control Theory*, Springer-Verlag, 1963

(Zurada 1997). Zurada, J. M., *Introduction to Artificial Neural Network*, Jaico Publishing House, Second Edition, 1997

VITA

Peter K. Ghavami received his BA from Oregon University in Mathematics with emphasis in Computer Science. He received his M.S. in Engineering Management from Portland State University. His career started as a software engineer, with progressive responsibilities at IBM Corp., Director of engineering, Chief Scientist, VP of Engineering and Product Management at various high technology firms. He was Director of Informatics at UW Medicine leading numerous clinical system implementations and new product development projects. He has been strategic advisor and acting VP of Informatics for various analytics companies.

He completed his PhD in Industrial and Systems Engineering at University of Washington, specializing in Prognostics, the application of analytics to predict failures in systems. He has authored several papers and book chapters on software process improvement, vector processing, distributed network architectures, and software quality. His first book, titled *Lean, Agile and Six Sigma Information Technology Management* was published in 2008. Peter is on the advisory board of several clinical analytics companies and often invited as lecturer and speaker on this topic. He is a member of IEEE Reliability Society, IEEE Life Sciences Initiative and HIMSS. He has been an active member of HIMSS and a contributor to the Data Analytics Task Force and a member of the HIMSS Clinical and Business Intelligence Committee.